AF851318

MENINGIOMAS – MANAGEMENT AND SURGERY

Edited by **Daniel Monleon**

Meningiomas – Management and Surgery
Edited by Daniel Monleon

Published by InTech

Janeza Trdine 9, 51000 Rijeka, Croatia

Copyright © 2012 InTech

All chapters are distributed under the Creative Commons Attribution 3.0 license, which allows users to download, copy and build upon published articles even for commercial purposes, as long as the author and publisher are properly credited, which ensures maximum dissemination and a wider impact of our publications. After this work has been published by InTech, authors have the right to republish it, in whole or part, in any publication of which they are the author, and to make other personal use of the work. Any republication, referencing or personal use of the work must explicitly identify the original source.

As for readers, this license allows users to download, copy and build upon published chapters even for commercial purposes, as long as the author and publisher are properly credited, which ensures maximum dissemination and a wider impact of our publications.

Notice

Statements and opinions expressed in the chapters are these of the individual contributors and not necessarily those of the editors or publisher. No responsibility is accepted for the accuracy of information contained in the published chapters. The publisher assumes no responsibility for any damage or injury to persons or property arising out of the use of any materials, instructions, methods or ideas contained in the book.

Publishing Process Manager Maja Kisic

Technical Editor Teodora Smiljanic

Cover Designer InTech Design Team

Additional hard copies can be obtained from orders@intechopen.com

Meningiomas – Management and Surgery, Edited by Daniel Monleon
p. cm.
978-953-51-0175-8

We are IntechOpen, the world's leading publisher of Open Access books

Built by scientists, for scientists

4,000+
Open access books available

116,000+
International authors and editors

120M+
Downloads

151
Countries delivered to

Our authors are among the
Top 1%
most cited scientists

12.2%
Contributors from top 500 universities

WEB OF SCIENCE™

Selection of our books indexed in the Book Citation Index in Web of Science™ Core Collection (BKCI)

Interested in publishing with us?
Contact book.department@intechopen.com

Numbers displayed above are based on latest data collected.
For more information visit www.intechopen.com

For EU product safety concerns:
IN TECH d.o.o., Prolaz Marije Krucifikse Kozulić 3, 51000 Rijeka, Croatia,
info@intechopen.com or visit our website at intechopen.com.

Meet the editor

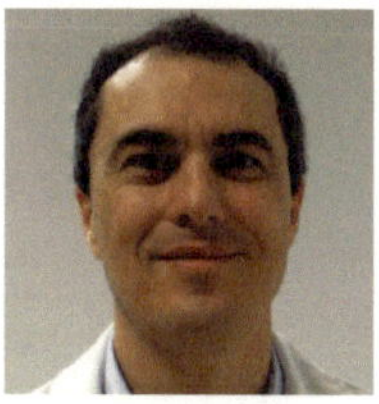

Dr Daniel Monleón is the Head of the Molecular Imaging and Metabolomics Lab, Fundación de Investigación del Hospital Clínico Universitario de Valencia, and Lecturer in Cell Biology at the Department of Pathology, University of Valencia, Spain. He has developed research for better understanding, classification and management of brain tumors for more than 10 years, publishing his works in the most prestigious journals in the field and receiving funds from the most competitive institutions, both at the national and international level. Dr Monleón is a member of the Editorial Board of several international peer-reviewed journals and was appointed as Scientific Manager of the European Coordinated Project eTUMOUR in 2004, aiming for a better classification of brain tumors based on their molecular properties. Dr Monleón is well known for developing multidisciplinary research integrating different expertise for a common goal.

Contents

Preface

The initial diagnosis of a brain tumour causes fear and insecurity in patients, their families and friends. The appropriate diagnosis, treatment and management requires the best skills that the neurosurgeons developed as a result of years of experience and research. The treatment of brain tumours, especially surgical, has improved greatly over the past decades. The ideal management involves many different techniques and expertise, even for the most benign forms.

Meningiomas are neoplasms that arise from the leptomeningeal covering of the brain and spinal cord, representing around one fourth of all Central Nervous System tumours. They are the second most common primary neoplasm of the central nervous system and display a remarkably wide spectrum of biological and histological properties. This heterogeneity has fascinated surgeons and pathologists since the word meningioma was first used by Harvey Cushing in 1922. Although the majority of these tumours are histologically benign, some meningiomas show signs of malignancy such as marked vascularity, loss of organoid structure, mitotic figures, nuclear pleomorphism, prominent nucleoli, focal necrosis, or infiltration to the adjacent brain. On the other hand, their positioning in the central nervous system can cause serious morbidity and/or mortality. The World Health Organization (WHO) classifies meningiomas into three histologic grades: Grade I (benign), Grade II (atypical), and Grade III (anaplastic), according to the clinical prognosis.

The management of patients with meningioma is usually a compromise between definitive removal of the tumor and minimization of neurologic damage. Initial management for patients with a benign meningioma typically consists of surgery, surgery plus radiation therapy, or radiation therapy alone. On the contrary, surgeons may choose to simply monitor patients showing asymptomatic or minimally symptomatic slow growing lesions for evidence of tumor growth, deferring initial treatment. In these cases, personalized follow-up schedules are of the utmost importance for proper patient management.

As a consequence, the most relevant aspects in the management of meningioma patients are therefore the surgical approach for initial treatment and a proper follow up strategy. During the preparation of this book, these aspects have been taken as primary targets in different chapters and sections. The book includes chapters dedicated to surgery, from neuronavigation to dural reconstruction, as well as those dedicated to management, including radiation therapy strategies and management of most malignant cases. We all think that the outcome is an extensive but focused manual that will be of high value during management of meningioma patient.

Dr. Daniel Monleon
Head of the Molecular Imaging and Metabolomics Lab of the Clinical Research Foundation, Hospital Clínico Universitario de Valencia,
Lecturer in Cell Biology at the Department of Pathology of the University of Valencia, Spain

Part 1

Management of Meningiomas

1

Management of Malignant Meningiomas

Danijela Levačić, David Nochlin, Thomas Steineke and Joseph C. Landolfi
JFK Brain Tumor Center, New Jersey Neuroscience Institute
USA

1. Introduction

Meningiomas are brain tumors that originate from arachnoid cap cells. They account for about one third of all brain tumors (CBTRUS, 2011), and their incidence increases with age. There are many histological subtypes of meningioma and they differ in their level of malignant behavior. The most commonly used World Health Organization (WHO) scheme (see 2.1) classifies them in three grades, which have distinct prognostic properties.

Malignant meningiomas (WHO grade III) are the most rare, but aggressive subtype of meningiomas. In comparison to other subtypes, they are understudied, likely due to their scarcity. The frequency of 1-3% among all intracranial meningiomas has been reported (Louis et al., 2007).

In this chapter, we are bringing a review of the available literature on malignant meningiomas. Because of the rarity of these tumors, patients with malignant meningiomas represent a very small part of any study population. Most studies analyze information on meningiomas of all subtypes, and the data on malignant ones had to be extracted from the larger population. In the lack of randomized clinical trials, these sporadic experiences and case reports became the foundation for the current clinical practices in diagnosis and treatment of patients with this rare disease. Our review includes the information on meningiomas in general, with focus on malignant meningiomas whenever specific data is available.

1.1 Frequency and Risk Factors

1.1.1 Hormonal Factors

Meningiomas in general are more common in women, with female predominance of 2-3 to 1, but this tendency diminishes in atypical and anaplastic meningiomas, in children and in radiation-induced meningiomas (Marosi et al.; Park & McLaren, 2009). Hormonal factors have been considered to play a role in this predominance.

A study on 125 women with meningiomas investigated the risk of meningiomas in relation to exogenous and endogenous sex hormones (Jhawar et al., 2003). The relative risk for premenopausal women was 2.48 and for postmenopausal women who received hormone therapy was 1.86. There was a nonsignificant increased risk of meningioma in parous as opposed to nulliparous women. The risk also trended up with increased BMI. No association was found for past or current use of oral contraceptives. The risk for meningiomas was increased among women exposed to either endogenous or exogenous sex hormones. However, an unexpected relationship with increase in age at menarche was also noted and remained unexplained.

Another study analyzed the relationship of exposure to female sex hormones and risk of brain tumors. It included 178 meningioma cases, 115 glioma cases and 323 controls (Wigertz et al., 2006). An increased relative risk of meningioma was found among postmenopausal women for ever use of hormone replacement therapy, with an odds ratio of 1.7. Women who had used long-acting hormonal contraceptives had an increased risk of meningioma. Hormone usage was not associated with glioma risk in this study. The findings suggest that the use of female sex steroids may increase the risk of meningioma.

A large retrospective review of data on 355,318 women evaluated for any medical issue (Blitshteyn et al. 2008) was done to investigate the association between meningioma and hormone replacement therapy (HRT). Five percent of this population (18,037 women) was documented as current or past HRT users. A positive correlation between diagnosis of meningioma and HRT use was found, with odds ratio of 2.2. The frequency of meningioma in women with either current or past HRT use was 865 in 100,000, whereas the frequency in women without the history of HRT use was 366 in 100,000. Therefore, HRT use may be a risk factor for meningioma.

1.1.2 Radiation

Radiation-induced meningiomas have a higher rate of multiplicity and atypia, compared to sporadic meningiomas (Park & McLaren, 2009). Historically, low doses of irradiation were used in treatment of tinea capitis until 1950s, and the analysis of data on 10,834 treated children showed the sevenfold increase in the incidence of meningioma, with latency period shorter with higher doses of irradiation (Ron et al., 1988). A strong dose-response relation was found, with the relative risk approaching 20 after estimated doses of approximately 2.5 Gy. Recurrences were more common in patients with radiation-induced meningiomas as compared to the sporadic.

Another study on childhood cancer survivors (Neglia et al., 2006) showed that meningiomas developed in 0.5% of patients treated with cranial irradiation, with median time of diagnosis 17 years after the diagnosis of original malignancy and the risk was directly related to the dose of cranial irradiation.

An increased incidence of meningiomas was found in survivors of the atomic bomb explosions in Japan. The incidence was higher with higher radiation doses and in people who were younger at the time of exposure (Park & McLaren, 2009).

1.1.3 Genetic Factors

There is also increased frequency of meningiomas in certain genetic diseases, like neurofibromatosis (NF type I and II) and familial meningioma. The association with other malignancies is suggestive of a common genetic basis.

Tumorigenesis of meningiomas involves activation of oncogenes and the loss of tumor suppressor genes. NF2 tumor suppressor gene has been found to be mutated in a large portion of meningiomas (Maxwell et al., 1998). Almost all cases of familial meningioma occur in association with NF2. The authors of a case report on two family members with spinal meningiomas, without any NF2 stigmata, conclude that a second tumor suppressor gene locus, other than NF2 acts in formation of familial sporadic meningioma. The conclusion is based on the presence of protein product merlin in specimens from both patients. Merlin has been implicated in the tumorigenesis of meningiomas.

1.1.4 Head Trauma

There is some suggestion of increased risk of meningioma following head trauma. A large case-control study (Preston-Martin et al., 1998) was done to investigate this suggestion based on prior case reports. It involved 1178 patients with gliomas and 330 with meningiomas, matched to 2236 controls. Risks of ever having experienced a head injury was highest for male patients with meningiomas (odds ratio = 1.5), but was lower for "serious" injuries. Latency of 15 to 24 years significantly increased the risk of meningioma among males. Odds ratios were lower for males with gliomas for any injury and in females in general. This has shown that the brain tumor risk after head trauma was strongest for meningiomas in men.

Another case-control study was conducted among women (Preston-Martin et al., 1980). One hundred-eighty-eight women with meningiomas were matched with their neighbors, and their experiences were compared. A history of head trauma was found to be associated with meningioma occurrence, with odds ratio of 2.0.

2. Histopathology

2.1 WHO Classification

Meningiomas are classified according to the World Health Organization (WHO) schema, which is based upon morphologic criteria. The latest, 2007 version of WHO classification divides meningiomas into 3 groups (Louis et al., 2007; Park et al., 2010):

- WHO grade I – Tumors that do not meet criteria for a higher grade lesion, based upon morphologic criteria. They are subdivided into: meningothelial, fibrous, transitional, psammomatous, angiomatous, microcystic, secretory, lymphoplasmacyte-rich and metaplastic. They are all considered to be of low risk for recurrence or aggressive growth and the treatment approach for all subtypes is the same.
- WHO grade II – Tumors with increased mitotic activity (≥4 mitoses per high powered field) and three or more of the following features: increased cellularity, small cells with a high nuclear/cytoplasmic ratio, prominent nucleoli, uninterrupted patternless or sheet-like growth, or foci of spontaneous or geographic necrosis. Subtypes include: atypical, chordoid and clear cell meningiomas. Alternative grading approaches identify individually scored parameters to arrive at a sum (Jääskeläinen et al., 1986; Louis et al., 2007), or simply combine hypercellularity with 5 or more mitoses per 10 high power fields.

- WHO grade III – Tumors with ≥20 mitoses per high-powered field and/or malignant characteristics resembling carcinoma, sarcoma or melanoma. Features that support the diagnosis of malignant meningioma include the loss of usual meningioma growth patterns, infiltration of underlying brain (Figure 1), abundant mitoses with atypical forms (Figure 2) and multifocal microscopic foci of necrosis (Figure 3). Subtypes include: papillary, rhabdoid and anaplastic (malignant) meningiomas. Although considered malignant, there are only isolated reports on any distant metastases. These tumors recur locally.

The WHO grading system has been revised over the years to better delineate the categories of patients with similar outcomes. With 2000/2007 classification, the differences in progression-free survival between histologic groups became significant, as compared to 1993. The major difference between 2000 and 2007 versions is that brain invasion became a criterion for classifying a meningioma as grade II or III, in a lesion that would otherwise be considered grade I.

Changes in classification criteria are to be considered when literature is reviewed, as they brought on a substantial shift with increasing the numbers of patients with WHO grade II tumors. The refined WHO criteria appear to be more accurate prognostically.

The likelihood of recurrence and/or aggressive behavior of meningioma increases with each higher grade. The proper classification of each tumor is very important in treatment planning. The tumors of lower grade can recur as a higher grade.

One hundred-sixteen patients were diagnosed with "malignant meningioma" (Perry et al., 1999) due to brain invasion, frank anaplasia (20 mitoses per 10 high-power fields or histology resembling carcinoma, sarcoma or melanoma) and/or extracranial metastasis. They were followed in a study, which concluded that histologic anaplasia, subtotal resection, 20 mitoses per 10 high-power fields and nuclear atypia were associated with poor survival. Survival time was highly variable, from 10 days to 24 years. Of 89 cases of meningioma that invaded the brain, 23% were otherwise benign, 61% were otherwise atypical and 17% were frankly anaplastic. Anaplastic meningiomas were usually fatal. Based on these findings it was suggested that the brain invasion constitutes an additional criterion for the diagnosis of atypical meningioma (WHO grade II), whereas frank anaplasia indicates high grade malignancy (WHO grade III)

2.2 Pathological Features

Papillary meningiomas are rare variant defined by the presence of perivascular pseudopapillary pattern in at least a part of the tumor. They tend to occur in children. Local invasion of the surrounding structures and invasion of the brain have been noted in 75% of these lesions, recurrence in 55% and metastasis in 20% (WHO, 2000).

Rhabdoid meningioma is an uncommon tumor containing patches or extensive sheets of rhabdoid cells, which are rounded tumor cells with eccentric nuclei, often with a prominent nucleolus, and prominent inclusion-like eosinophilic cytoplasm comprised of whorled intermediate filaments. Most rhabdoid meningiomas have high proliferative indices and additional histological features of malignancy (WHO, 2000).

Anaplastic (malignant) meningiomas are tumors exhibiting histological features of frank malignancy far in excess of the abnormalities present in atypical meningiomas. This includes either obviously malignant cytology or a high mitotic index (≥20 mitoses per 10 high-power fields) (WHO, 2000). They are found to have a high proliferation rate as well (Figure 4).

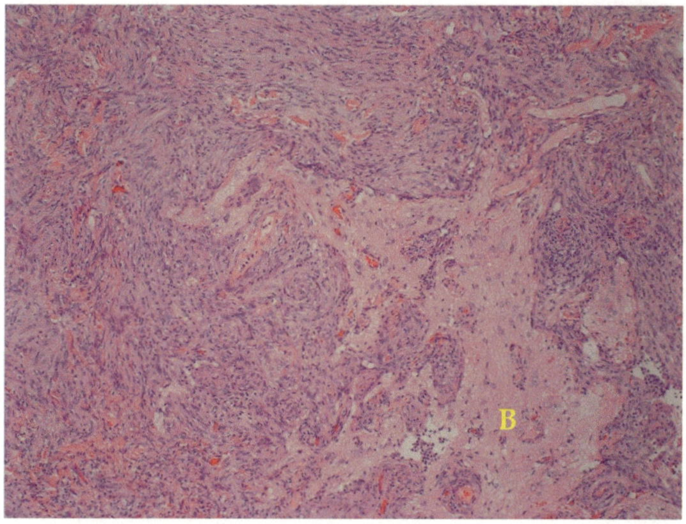

Fig. 1. Brain (B) Invasion. H&E, X10 (original magnification)

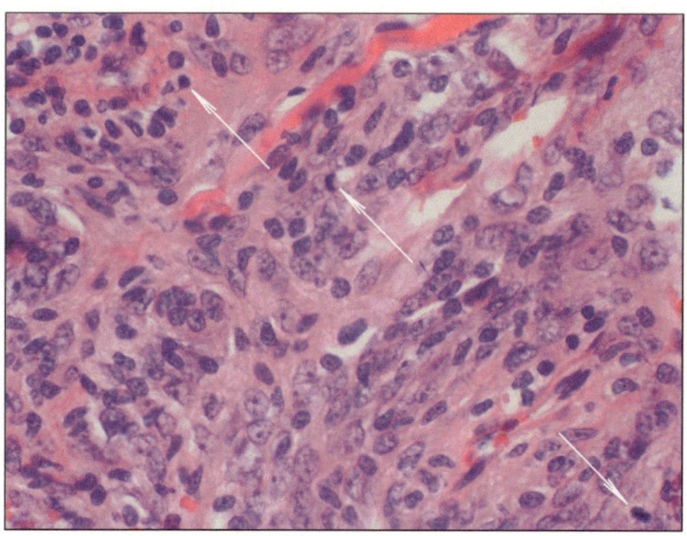

Fig. 2. Mitoses (white arrows). H&E, X60 (original magnification)

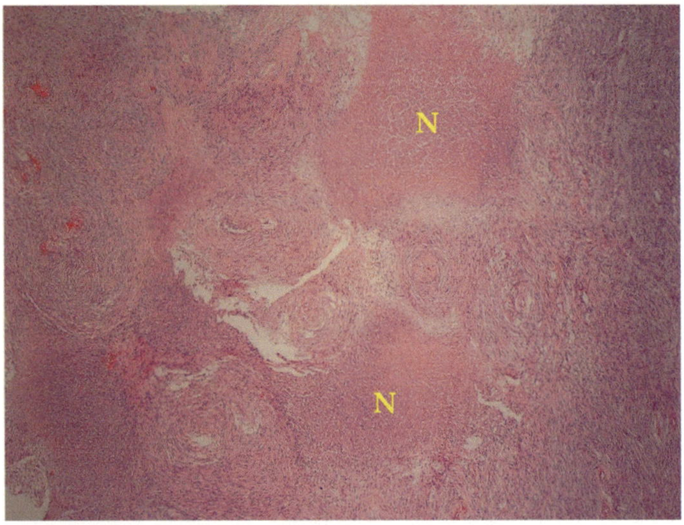

Fig. 3. Necrosis (N). H&E, X4 (original magnification)

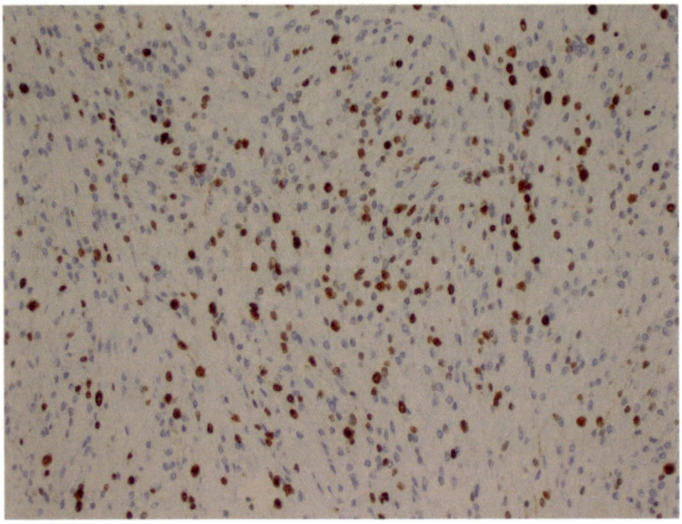

Fig. 4. High proliferation index. Ki67 (MIB-1) cell proliferation marker. Immunohistochemistry. DAKO Envision Flex+ with or without heat induced epitope retrieval techniques. X20 (original magnification)

3. Imaging Characteristics

Diagnostic process on patients with intracranial masses typically starts with brain imaging, after the initial clinical assessment. Oftentimes, intracranial masses can be incidental findings on the imaging done for unrelated reasons, such as work-up for head trauma. The most common clinical scenario is a finding of suspicious lesion on a plain computed tomography (CT), which is then followed by gadolinium enhanced magnetic resonance imaging (MRI).

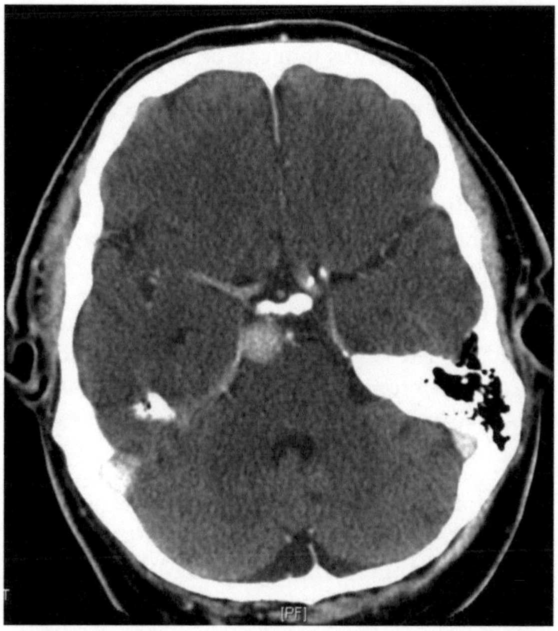

Fig. 5. Contrast enhanced CT image of clival meningioma in a 69-year-old man. Dural tail is visible.

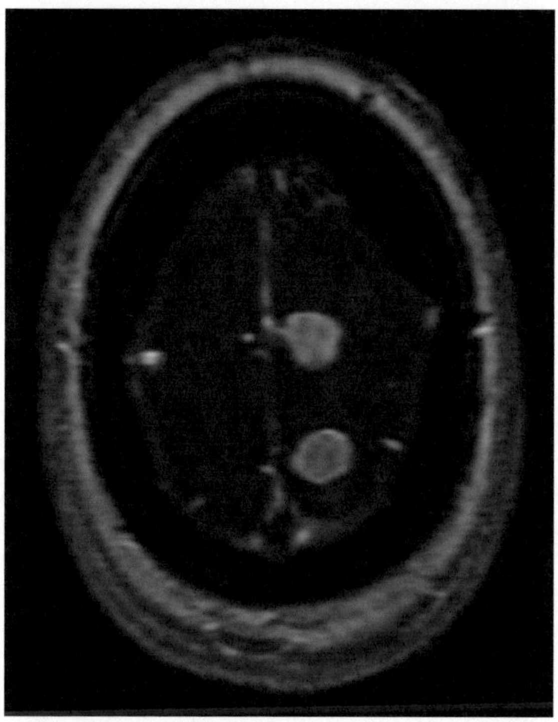

Fig. 6. Axial T1 MRI with gadolinium of the left sided convexity meningiomas in a 62-year old woman. Anterior lesion has visible dural tail.

This applies to meningiomas as well. Although a definitive diagnosis cannot be made solely based on imaging, there are some features that can be suggestive of meningiomas.

The most common locations for meningiomas (in descending order) are in parasagittal dura, convexities, sphenoid wing, cerebellopontine angle cistern, olfactory groove and planum sphenoidale. Ninety percent occur supratentorially. One percent of meningiomas occur outside the CNS, presumably from embryologic arachnoid rests. Because meningiomas arise from arachnoid cap cells, they can occur anywhere that arachnoid exists (Grossman & Yousem, 2003)

The grade of tumor cannot be determined based on imaging, but the benign lesions tend to appear as well demarcated, ovoid extradural masses. With increase in tumor grade, the lesions tend to lose their sharp contours, often demonstrating invasion of surrounding brain tissue, bone and/or venous sinuses. Necrotic centers and calcified portions can be seen as well.

A retrospective study on 75 patients who underwent intracranial meningioma resection was done to determine correlation between aggressive imaging features and advanced histopathological grade in meningiomas (Hsu et al., 2010). Six aggressive imaging features were evaluated: intratumoral cystic change, hyperostosis of the adjacent skull, bony destruction, extracranial tumor extension through the skull base foramina, arterial encasement and peritumoral brain edema. Fifty-nine tumors were classified as benign, according to WHO classification, and 16 as atypical/malignant. Only intratumoral cystic change and extracranial tumor extension through the skull base foramina were more prevalent in atypical/malignant meningiomas.

"Dural tail" is highly characteristic of meningioma and it has been seen in up to 72% of the cases (Grossman & Yousem, 2003). The dura is trailing off away from the lesion in crescentic fashion (Figures 5 & 6).

The degree of parenchymal edema is variable in meningiomas, and it is not necessarily proportionate to their size. It seems to correlate with location, because meningiomas adjacent to cerebral cortex tend to incite greater edema than those along the basal cisterns or planum. It may be caused by compressive ischemia, venous stasis, aggressive growth or parasitization of pial vessels (Grossman & Yousem, 2003).

Bony changes associated with meningiomas may be hyperostotic or osteolytic and occur in 20% to 46% of cases (44). They can be suggestive of malignant behavior, but the hyperostosis along the inner table only can be just the reactive changes rather than neoplastic invasion. Secondary bone involvement occurs in up to 50% of skull base meningiomas. It is uncommon in convexity tumors (Park & McLaren, 2009).

3.1 Magnetic Resonance Imaging (MRI)

MRI is preferred in imaging meningiomas, as it is superior in demonstrating dural origin, as well as vascularity, edema, sinus and bone invasion. Meningiomas are typically isointense or hypointense to gray matter on T1 and isointense or hyperintense on T2 weighted images (Figure 7). They enhance with gadolinium, but they might have areas of necrosis and calcification, which do not enhance.

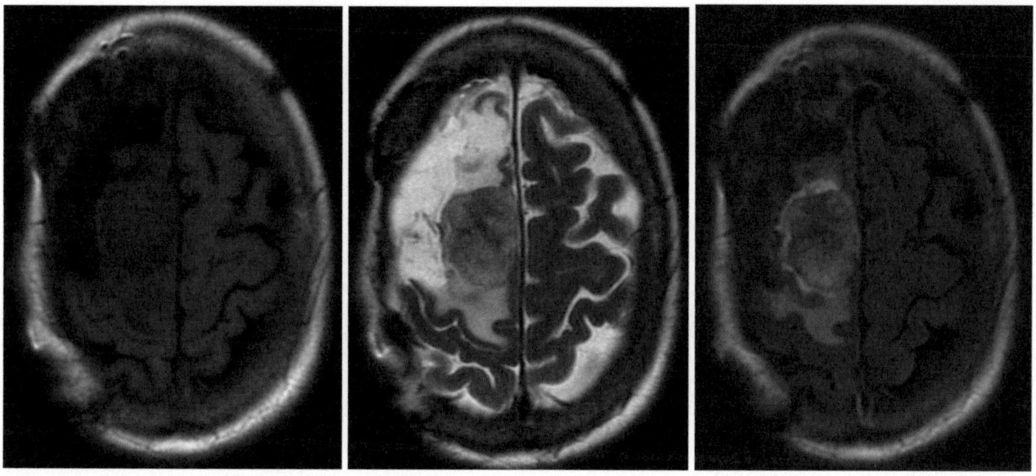

Fig. 7. Axial MRI of a right parasagittal anaplastic meningioma in a 72-year-old woman. Image on the left is FLAIR T1, in the middle is T2 and on the right is T2 FLAIR with gadolinium.

3.2 Computed Tomography (CT)

CT scans typically show well-defined, smooth-contoured extra-axial mass, which displaces the normal brain tissue. Sometimes meningiomas can be multilobulated or calcified. They can be isointense with the normal brain tissue, but they enhance uniformly with the intravenous contrast administration, making the diagnosis easier. This is more typical of benign meningiomas.

Characteristics suggestive of aggressive behavior (Figure 8) of the tumor are: indistinct margins, marked edema, mushroom-like projections from tumor, deep brain parenchymal infiltration and heterogenous enhancement (Shapir et al., 1985 as cited in Park & McLaren, 2009).

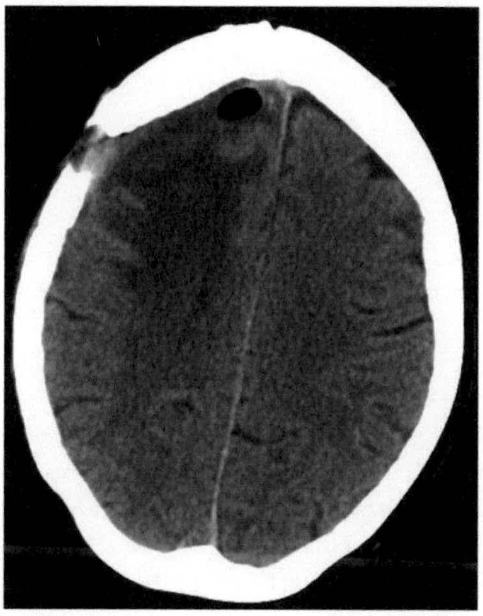

Fig. 8. CT image of a right parasagittal anaplastic meningioma in a 69-year-old woman (same patient as in Figure 7, three years earlier)

3.3 Positron Emission Tomography (PET)

PET is not routinely used in diagnostics of meningiomas, but it has its place in diagnostics of malignant meningiomas, considering that it can help predict aggressiveness of a meningioma and the potential for recurrence (Di Chiro et al., 1987; Park & McLaren, 2009).

3.4 Angiography

Angiography was used more often prior to development of MRI and CT techniques. Findings of arterial supply from meningeal vessels and the delayed vascular blush were helpful in diagnosis of meningiomas. They have both dural and pial supply. Angiography is now mainly used as part of the pre-operative embolization procedures.

4. Treatment

The National Comprehensive Cancer Network® (NCCN®) guidelines summarize the contemporary approach to meningioma management (NCCN®, 2011):

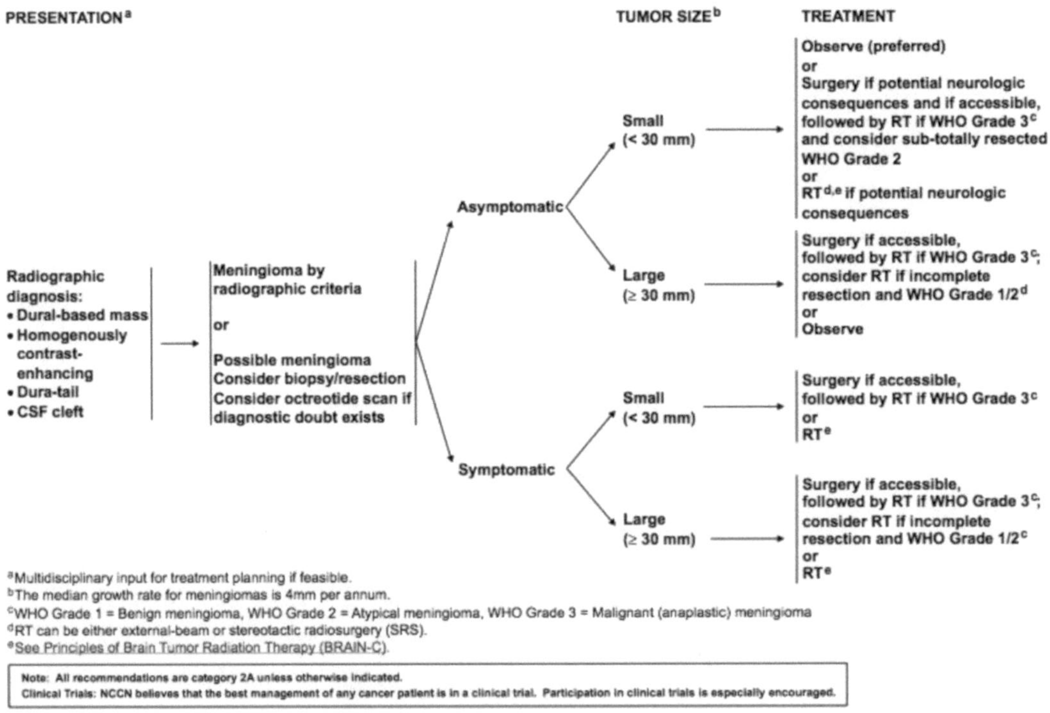

Reproduced with permission from the NCCN Clinical Practice Guidelines in Oncology (NCCN Guidelines™) for Central Nervous System Cancers V.2.2011. © 2011 National Comprehensive Cancer Network, Inc. All rights reserved. The NCCN Guidelines™ and illustrations herein may not be reproduced in any form for any purpose without the express written permission of the NCCN. To view the most recent and complete version of the NCCN Guidelines, go online to NCCN.org. NATIONAL COMPREHENSIVE CANCER NETWORK®, NCCN®, NCCN GUIDELINES™, and all other NCCN Content are trademarks owned by the National Comprehensive Cancer Network, Inc.

This subchapter contains the review of available literature on various modalities of treatment supplemented with experiences from our own institution. The existing data on therapy most commonly comes from retrospective studies on patients with all types of meningiomas, with only small subgroups having malignant forms. The lack of hard evidence on efficacy of different treatment approaches makes it difficult to standardize the treatment algorithm for malignant meningioma. However, the general consensus is that surgical resection, as radical as possible, should be performed. If indicated, a pre-operative embolization should be done a day before resection. Radiation therapy following surgery is found to be beneficial, and therefore it became a standard of care for these patients. Various modalities of systemic therapy have been tried, mostly on patients who have exhausted all primary options, but unfortunately, their efficacy has not been very promising so far.

4.1 Embolization

As malignant meningiomas are highly vascular tumors, preoperative embolization can make them more resectable. It is most applied to skull base meningiomas, a day prior to surgery (Carli et al., 2010; Matsuda et al., 2011; Oka et al., 1998; Rosen et al., 2002).

Again, the information on malignant meningiomas alone is very scarce. Available sources provide information on meningiomas in general.

A retrospective analysis on 167 cranial base meningiomas (Rosen et al., 2002), which were embolized showed that a good to excellent embolization was achieved in 91% of patients, without permanent neurological sequelae. Cranial base meningiomas were defined as tumors originating from olfactory groove, tuberculum sellae, medial sphenoid wing, petro-clival region or foramen magnum. In 20 patients, embolization was not attempted due to the risk of new neurologic deficits or lack of an appropriate vessel for embolization. Fifteen patients (9%) experienced permanent neurologic deficits or medical morbidity as a result of embolization. The conclusion of this study points out that the benefits of embolization as an adjunct to cranial base surgery have to be weighted against the morbidity that comes with this procedure.

Another study involving 20 patients with skull-base meningiomas (Oka et al., 1998) revealed significantly smaller blood loss during surgical resection in patients who underwent pre-operative embolization. This only applied to tumors smaller than 6 cm. There was no difference in blood loss in tumors larger than 6 cm, perhaps because larger meningiomas tend to have tiny blood vessels that are unsuitable for pre-operative embolization. There was no difference in the length of surgery between the embolized and non-embolized group. However, the embolized group tended to show better clinical outcome.

The risks of widely used particle embolization (Carli et al., 2010) were analyzed on 198 patients (201 meningiomas). Indications for embolization were: pre-operative in 165 meningiomas, adjunctive to radiosurgery in 8 and sole therapy in 28. Complications were defined as any neurologic deficits or death that occurred during or after embolization. They occurred in 11 patients (5.6%); 10 were hemorrhagic and 1 ischemic. Complications of embolization resulted in death of 2 and dependency in 5 patients. The use of small particles (45-150 μm) was the only risk factor for complications. With the complication rate of 5.6% and the increased risks with small particles, the use of small polyvinyl alcohol particles is not recommended.

Another study (Matsuda et al., 2011) assessed the atypical and ischemic features of embolized meningiomas, comparing 29 patients that underwent pre-operative embolization with 29 who did not. Large polyvinyl alcohol particles (150-250 μm) were used for embolization via middle meningeal or occipital artery, until the stagnation of the contrast agent in the feeding artery was accomplished. The embolization material was invisible in tumors and the large particles were believed to remain in the feeding vessels. Small cells, clear cells, rhabdoid-like cells and pseudopapillary pattern were thought to be associated with embolization using the large particles, instead of development of necrosis. There were no complications of the embolization procedure. Embolization was done 3 to 355 hours before the surgical extirpation. The two groups of patients had no significant differences in gender, age, tumor location and reoccurrence or regrowth of tumor. However, the differences in histopathological features between the two groups were evident. They included higher mitotic activity, brain invasion, increased cellularity, prominent nucleoli, small cells with high nuclear/cytoplasmic ratio, sheet-like growth and geographic necrosis. Even more evident differences were noted in occurrence of cytoplasmic vacuoles, intercellular discohesion and perivascular cuffs. In accordance to WHO 2007 classification, 11 patients (38%) in embolized group were classified as grade II atypical meningioma, versus 7 patients (24%) in non-embolized group. There were no patients with anaplastic (grade III) meningiomas. It appears that the increased frequency of atypical features in pre-operatively embolized meningiomas could lead to prognostic inaccuracies and overly aggressive therapy. However, the possibility of patient selection bias rather than embolization artifacts leading to higher number of atypical meningiomas in embolized group cannot be excluded, especially considering a rather small patient sample. Proliferative activity in embolized meningiomas does not always reflect genuine tumor proliferation and should not be used to assess malignancy. Ischemic histologic features (including small cells with high N/C ratios, cytoplasmic vacuoles, intercellular discohesion and perivascular cuffs) were identified in embolized meningiomas. Therefore, histological findings and determination of grading should be evaluated cautiously in the cases of embolized meningiomas.

4.2 Surgical Options

Complete surgical resection, including its dural attachement is a preferred therapeutic approach for all meningiomas, including malignant. As delineated in NCCN Guidelines (NCCN, 2011; see above), surgery is the first line of treatment for all symptomatic and for large asymptomatic meningiomas. As meningiomas are highly vascular, pre-operative embolization is often used (see 4.1). With advances of modern imaging techniques, microsurgery and image-guided intraoperative approaches, this can be achieved in most tumors at accessible locations, minimizing the damage to normal brain tissue. However, malignant meningiomas often cannot be completely resected. Subtotal resection is then combined with radiation therapy (see 4.3). The extent of surgery is balanced with minimizing neurological deficits possibly caused by resection. Complete resection is usually attempted for tumors of the convexity, olfactory groove, anterior third of the sagittal sinus and some tentorial and posterior fossa tumors. Posterior sagittal region or clivus are less accessible, thus commonly allowing for partial resection, which is then followed by radiation therapy. Tumors involving medial sphenoid wing or cavernous sinus are deemed inaccessible, and surgery is generally not attempted.

4.2.1 Extent of Resection and Tendency for Recurrence

The extent of surgical resection is described with Simpson grading system (Simpson, 1957), still widely accepted since its publication:

- Grade I - Macroscopically complete removal of the tumor, with excision of its dural attachment and of any abnormal bone. Includes resection of venous sinus, if involved.
- Grade II - Macroscopically complete removal of the tumor and of its visible extensions, with coagulation of its dural attachment.
- Grade III - Macroscopically complete removal of the intradural tumor, without resection or coagulation of its dural attachment or its extradural extensions (e.g. an invaded sinus or hyperostotic bone).
- Grade IV - Partial removal, leaving intradural tumor in situ.
- Grade V - Simple decompression, with or without biopsy.

The author (Simpson, 1957) analyzed the post-operative results of two series of patients, one of 235 cases (operated on in Oxford, from 1938 to 1954) and one of 97 cases (London, from 1928 to 1938). A system of grading according to the scope of resection was presented and applied to those cases, 265 in all, surviving more than six months. Following 90 operations of grade I, there were 8 recurrences (9%). Following 114 grade II resections, there were 18 recurrences (19%, with cases treated within the last 5 years of study period being excluded). These recurrences became apparent after an average period of five years. Long-delayed recurrences, though clearly possible, appeared unusual. After incomplete resections, grades III-V, the incidence of symptomatic recurrence was naturally much greater, but a number of patients treated by limited excisions were given long periods of relief. In this study, the author emphasized that in the clinical sense, meningiomas may be benign, locally invasive or frankly malignant. The frequency of local infiltration of venous sinuses was found in 15% of cases, infiltration of bone in 20% and of brain in 3.7%. Haematogenous metastasis was found in two patients.

Though this study was conducted more than a half century ago, its general observations are still considered relevant and the new data is only confirming them. Simpson grading system for the extent of surgery is commonly used today in its original form. However, some authors propose adding grade 0 to it (Borovich et al., 1986), entailing a wide resection of the dura around the attachment zone of the meningioma.

More contemporary data reflect the advances of modern surgical techniques and overall medical treatment. Publications regarding malignant meningiomas specifically are still scarce and the few existing studies are retrospective. They all do point to the increased benefit of surgery followed by radiotherapy. With the lack of prospective studies on the use of post-operative radiotherapy for malignant meningiomas, it has nevertheless come to represent the standard of care at most institutions (Hanft et al., 2010).

One retrospective study of 38 patients with 48 malignant meningioma resections (28 total and 20 subtotal) was done to determine the time to recurrence, among other parameters (Dziuk et al., 1998). Twenty-five lesions were treated at initial presentation and 23 were treated as recurrent disease (13 had transformed from previously benign meningiomas). Nineteen patients received post-operative radiation therapy. Histological subtypes included 32 anaplastic meningiomas, 11 hemangiopericytomas, 2 meningiosarcomas and 3 papillary meningiomas. One patient presented with multicentric disease, and 4 had multicentric disease at recurrence. Tumors were located on frontal/parietal convexity in 33%, falx/parasagittal sinus in 26%, temporal convexity in 10%, tentorium and posterior fossa in 5% each, and in occipital convexity, sphenoid wing, olfactory groove, tuberculum sellae and foramen magnum in 3% of lesions per each location. Eight percent of patients had lesions at multiple sites. Follow-up ranged from 3 to 144 months, with 5 patients excluded from analysis. Disease free survival (DFS) at 24 months for all patients was 74%, and at 5 years it was 25%. DFS at 5 years was 39% following total resection versus 0% after subtotal resection. For all totally resected lesions, the 5-year DFS was improved from 28% for surgery alone to 57% with adjuvant radiotherapy. As there were no distant failures, local control was equated to actuarial DFS. Twenty out of 26 surgery alone meningiomas recurred, as did 7 of 17 receiving adjuvant radiotherapy. Combined results for surgery with and without adjuvant radiation revealed the following: When analyzed by extent of resection, there was a trend to increased DFS at 24 months, 80% for total resection versus 66% for subtotal resection. It was significant at 5 years, with 39% versus 0%. Initially treated lesions displayed a higher rate of local control versus recurrent lesions, with a 5-year DFS of 33% versus 19% respectively. Totally excised lesions treated with surgery alone had 5-year DSF of 28%, compared to 0% for the subtotally excised lesions. The 5-year DFS of surgery alone patients was essentially the same for initial versus recurrent resections. However, the median time to local failure was significantly longer for initial versus recurrent disease, 43.5 months versus 18 months, respectively.

Recurring lesions have an increased tendency toward multicentricity, and multicentric lesions have an increased tendency for recurrence. Once disease has recurred, there is an increased probability for a subsequent local failure, and the disease/progression-free interval is shortened (Salazar, 1988 as cited in Dziuk et al., 1998).

Probability for local control was once again shown to be dependent upon the extent of resection. The meningioma location impacts the potential for total resection: the most accessible convexity lesions are completely resected in 96% of cases, parasagittal/falx tumors 80%, olfactory groove 70%, sphenoid ridge 50%, tuberculum sellae 48% and posterior fossa 43% (Salazar, 1988 as cited in Dziuk et al., 1998). However, total resectability by location does not translate into decreased recurrence by location: the parassagittal region is commonly reported to have the highest recurrence rate. The difference is presumed due to the resection of as little dura as possible in the meningiomas of the middle and posterior sagittal sinus to avoid occlusion.

The tendency of meningiomas to recur even after they appeared to the naked eye as completely surgically removed (Simpson grade I) is attributed in some cases to malignancy and more commonly to an erroneous belief that the excision was total (Borovich & Doron, 1986). In a study on 14 patients with globular meningiomas (Borovich & Doron, 1986), authors examined the dura mater around the meningiomas for evidence of regional multifocality. Meningotheliomatous cell aggregates were demonstrated in 100% of dural strips, which were removed from the line of attachment of each globular meningioma. The cell aggregates were in the form of dural clusters or nodes protruding from the inner aspect of the dura. They appeared benign. Control strips of convexity dura mater taken from 10 neurosurgical patients without meningioma failed to show these meningotheliomatous conglomerates. These findings indicate that solitary globular meningiomas represent only the most visible growth in the midst of a neoplastic field change spreading over a wide area of dura mater.

Regional multiplicity in meningiomas would thus seem to be rule (Borovich et al., 1986). The authors of this study proposed dividing recurrences after grade I resections into true local and false regional. A local recurrence would be defined as a regrowth within the limits of the previous dural flap. Regional recurrence would be the new growth outside the previous craniotomy site, which should not be considered as a recurrence but as a new primary site. With the idea that a wider resection of the dura around the attachment zone of the meningioma would reduce the incidence of recurrence, the authors proposed adding Simpson grade 0 to the existing classification, defining more radical total resection.

In a large cohort study (Sughrue et al., 2010) of 63 patients with WHO grade III meningiomas, all the patients underwent post-operative radiation therapy after the primary surgery and they were followed for median time of 5 years. Fifty-eight percent of those patients who underwent a second surgery for recurrent meningioma received either ^{125}I brachytherapy implants or gamma-knife radiosurgery. Nearly 50% of patients had radiographic recurrence. The 2-, 5- and 10-year overall survival rates following initial surgery were 82, 61 and 40%, respectivelly. There was a significant survival benefit with repeat surgery for recurrent meningiomas (median survival of 53 months versus 25 months). Interestingly, patients treated with near-total resection experienced improved overall survival when compared with patients treated with gross-total resection at initial and repeat operations. Twelve (19%) of 63 patients experienced significant neurological morbidity referable to the resection of their tumors.

4.2.2 Surgical Morbidity and Mortality

The reported incidence of neurologic deficits as a direct complication of surgery ranges from 2 to 30%, depending on the location of the tumor and the extent of resection. Cortical brain injury may occur if the arachnoid and pia are adherent to the tumor and the pial vasculature is disrupted. Surgeries for skull base meningiomas pose risk for cranial nerve deficits.

The reports on overall surgical mortality vary with patient selection, as well as with changes in surgical care.

The cumulative observed survival rate of 935 patients who underwent surgery for intracranial meningioma (operated on between 1953 and 1980) was 91% at 3 months, 89% at 1 year and 63% at 15 years (Kallio et al., 1992). Significant risk factors for operative mortality (7%) for the 652 patients (operated on from 1966 to 1980) were poor preoperative clinical condition, absence of epilepsy, old age, incomplete tumor removal, pulmonary embolism and intracranial hematoma requiring evacuation. In 828 patients who survived the first post-operative year, the excess risk of death for up to 15 years was related to incomplete tumor removal, poor pre- and post-operative clinical condition, anaplasia of the tumor and hyperostosis. Patients with partial resections had a 4.2-fold relative excess risk of death as compared to patients with complete resections of tumors. Also, patients with malignant tumors had a 4.6-fold risk as compared with those who had benign tumors.

The higher mortality in older age population can be found in many older reports. However, the advances in surgical techniques as well as a careful selection of surgical candidates among the elderly have the potential of changing this picture. A retrospective study on 17 patients who underwent surgery for intracranial meningioma in their 9th decade of life (Mastronardi et al., 1995) showed that severe systemic disease and functional limitations had a major post-operative morbidity and mortality. The risk of post-operative morbidity was higher when the maximum diameter of the tumor was >5 cm.

4.2.3 Peri-operative Management

Seizures can be the sole symptom at the initial presentation of patients with meningioma, as well as the part of the more complex presentation. They can also occur post-operatively. Prophylaxis with anticonvulsant medications prior to surgery in patients who never had seizures is not indicated. Post-operative prophylaxis on patients undergoing resections of supratentorial tumors is indicated, with gradual tapering and discontinuing the medication in patients who had no seizures.

Cerebral edema is managed with administration of corticosteroids, which are post-surgically tapered if clinically feasible.

Deep venous thrombosis (DVT) appears to be especially problematic in patients with meningiomas, both because of the generally increased risks of DVT in patients undergoing any brain surgery and because meningiomas can produce hypercoagulable state. In 46 patients who underwent brain tumor resections, the incidence of DVT was 72% for meningioma patients, 60% for glioblastoma patients and 20% for brain metastasis patients (Sawaya et al., 1992). There was no correlation between the occurrence of DVT and the "usual suspects" among the risk factors for DVT. This finding, along with the marked variation in the incidence of DVT between the different brain tumor groups, strongly suggests that bilological factors play more important role than clinical factors in developing post-operative thrombosis. Pre-operative hemostatic profile was further investigated on 42 brain tumor patients (Sawaya & Glas-Greenwalt, 1992) and the occurrence of DVT was found to be higher with increased prothrombin time, plasminogen and total fibrinolytic activity and with decreased fibrinogen level. This overall trend in the group of patients with DVT after brain tumor resection lead to the conclusion that this hemostatic disorder is most closely related to a subclinical form of chronic disseminated intravascular coagulation syndrome. Pneumatic compression boots and prophylactic anticoagulation post-operatively for all patients with brain tumors should be considered.

4.3 Radiation Therapy

Radiation therapy is used in addition to subtotal surgical resection of meningiomas, as a sole therapy for unresectable tumors and oftentimes for completely resected tumors with high risk of recurrence per their histopathological features. Like with other therapeutic modalities used for the treatment of meningioma, there are no randomized trials providing evidence of its efficacy and safety. The available observational studies uniformly show the improvement in progression-free survival of patients who received radiation as compared to those who did not.

4.3.1 Effectiveness of Radiation Therapy

There is no general agreement on the use of radiation for partially removed tumors immediately after the initial surgery or upon the development of recurrence. Just like in surgical therapy, the techniques in radiation therapy have significantly improved overtime. The improvement of imaging techniques have contributed to better results as well.

This was clearly shown in a retrospective analysis of 140 patients who received radiation therapy as an adjuvant to subtotal resection of intracranial meningiomas, from 1967 to 1990 (Goldsmith et al., 1994). Of 140 meningiomas, 117 were benign and 23 were malignant. The overall survival rate at 5 years was 85% for the benign and 58% for the malignant tumor groups; the 5-year progression-free survival (PFS) rates were 89% and 48%, respectively. The 10-year overall and PFS rates for patients with benign meningiomas was 77%. Improvement in this rate was not related to tumor size, but to a younger age and treatment after 1980 (when CT and MRI became available for planning therapy). Prior to 1980, the radiation therapy volumes were based exclusively upon the surgeon's assessment of the site and volume of residual disease. Availability of CT and/or MRI allowed for incorporating more precise information about the residual tumor into the radiation planning. The 5-year PFS rate for patients with benign meningiomas treated after 1980 was 98% versus 77% for patients treated before 1980. Survival also improved with increasing the minimum radiation dose. None of these factors affected the survival rates of patients with malignant meningiomas.

The objective of the study on 101 patients with skull base meningiomas was to analyze long-term local control and complications after radiotherapy (Mendenhall et al., 2003). Sixty-six patients were treated with radiotherapy alone and 35 were treated with radiotherapy after subtotal surgical resection. Sixty-one patients had previously untreated tumors and 40 had tumors that recurred after prior surgery. The long-term local control rates were 95% at 5 years, 92% at 10 years and 92% at 15 years. The probability of long-term progression-free survival after radiotherapy exceeded 90% and was comparable to the results of complete resection and radiosurgery.

The effectiveness of radiotherapy was assessed in a retrospective study of 119 patients with atypical (69%) or malignant (31%) meningiomas treated with external beam radiotherapy (EBRT) after initial complete resection in 94 cases and for recurrence in 25 patients (Pasquier et al., 2008). The overall survival rates at 5 and 10 years were 65% and 51%, respectively. They were influenced by age over 60 years, low Karnofski performance status and high mitotic rate. The 5- and 10-year disease-free survival rates were 58% and 48%, respectively and were significantly affected by Karnofski performance status and high mitotic rate.

In a study on 936 primary intracranial meningiomas (Jääskeläinen et al., 1986), 94.3% were histologically benign (WHO grade I), 4.7% were atypical (grade II) and 1% were anaplastic (grade III). Only 26% of atypical or anaplastic meningiomas appeared completely innocent on a CT scan. Five years after complete removal, the recurrence rate was 3% for benign meningiomas, 38% for atypical and 78% for anaplastic ones. In spite of post-operative radiotherapy, four out of five anaplastic meningiomas recurred. This data supports the widely accepted practice of using radiation as adjuvant therapy for meningiomas of WHO grade II and III even after gross total resection, due to the increased rate of recurrence of these tumors, even though the effectiveness for malignant meningiomas specifically appears modest.

Previously cited analysis of 38 patients with malignant meningiomas, 19 of which received post-operative radiotherapy (Dziuk et al., 1998, see 4.2.1), showed that the adjuvant radiation following initial resection increased the 5-year disease-free survival (DFS) rates from 15% to 80%. When administered for recurrent lesions, adjuvant radiotherapy improved the 2-year DFS from 50% to 89%, but had no impact on 5-year DFS. Multivariate analysis indicated that the extent of resection, adjuvant radiotherapy and recurrence status were independent prognostic factors.

4.3.2 Dosage and Toxicity

The authors of the above-mentioned study (Dziuk et al., 1998) also pointed out the importance of treatment volume, recommending 3-4 cm margins around the pre-operative tumor volume. The dose response was established, with recommendation of 60 Gy at conventional fractionation. The adjuvant radiotherapy for the 9 subtotally resected lesions in this study did not provide long-term benefit, but 7 of them received 54 Gy or less.

The importance of radiation dose is illustrated by a retrospective series of 140 patients with benign or malignant meningiomas (Goldsmith et al., 1994), as described above (see 4.3.1). Of 117 patients with benign meningiomas, those treated with doses >52 Gy had better 10-year survival (93% versus 65% with ≤52 Gy). Similarly, among the patients with malignant meningiomas, the 5-year progression-free survival was better with doses >54 Gy (63% versus 17% with doses ≤ 53 Gy).

Available literature uniformly recognizes the increased efficacy of radiotherapy that comes with the increased doses, which of course, has to be balanced with the risks of injury for surrounding tissue. There is, however, little variation on recommended dose. Per (Park et al., 2010), when radiation therapy is applied post-operatively for residual disease, a dose of 54 Gy is used in daily fractions of 1.8 to 2 Gy for benign meningiomas. Atypical and anaplastic meningiomas are treated with higher doses, typically 59.4 Gy.

The recommended dose of adjuvant radiotherapy for best long-term control per (Dziuk et al., 1998) is 60 Gy (especially for subtotally resected disease) and it should be administered simultaneously with an initial complete resection. A 4 cm margin for the initial 50 Gy is advised.

4.3.3 Types of Radiotherapy

The goal of any type of radiation therapy is to deliver maximum dose of radiation to the lesion, while sparing the surrounding viable tissue. The commonly used techniques are stereotactic radiosurgery (SRS), stereotactic radiotherapy (SRT) and intensity-modulated radiation therapy (IMRT) (50). There is some preliminary data on proton beam therapy, which might be useful. Boron neutron capture therapy (BNCT) was tried on two patients, one of whom had anaplastic meningioma (Aiyama et al., 2011). The conclusion was that BNCT could be a safe palliative therapy for malignant brain tumors.

SRS utilizes multiple convergent beams to deliver a high single dose of radiation to a radiographically discrete treatment volume, thereby minimizing injury to adjacent structures (Park et al., 2010b). It is used for tumors in close proximity to critical structures (ex. optic nerve). Radiation alone can be also used for tumors in inaccessible locations like cavernous sinus or medial sphenoid wing. The most well-known machine used is Gamma-Knife®, utilizing cobalt-60. It is best used on lesions of ≤ 3.5 cm in size. The typical dose used to treat meningiomas is 12-14 Gy to the 50% Isodose line. This is done at a single sitting.

SRT is similar to SRS, using focused radiation, only fractionated over a series of sessions (Park et al., 2010b). Fractionation improves normal tissue tolerance of radiation, so SRT may be a reasonable alternative for patients with surgically inaccessible lesions. These machines are linear accelerator based and they are more suitable for use on tumors > 3.5 cm in size. The most common machines are CyberKnife® and Novalis Tx®.

IMRT relies upon software and modification of standard linear accelerator output to vary the radiation intensity across each treatment field (Park et al., 2010b). Similarly to SRS and SRT, it is useful for targets juxtaposed to radiation-sensitive structures. It is also particularly valuable for treatment of lesions with complex shape, such as those involving the skull base.

4.4 Systemic Treatment

Despite advances in surgery, radiation therapy and radio-surgery, there remains a small but important subset of patients with meningiomas who develop recurrent disease refractory to conventional therapies. To date, chemotherapies have shown minimal activity and hormonal therapies have proven to be largely ineffective. Progress in identifying alternative forms of therapy for these patients has been limited by poor understanding of the molecular pathogenesis of meningiomas and the critical molecular changes driving tumor growth, and by the lack of meningioma cell lines and tumor models for preclinical studies (Wen et al., 2010).

Most data is collected from observational studies, and unfortunately, none of the agents have proven efficacy in progression-free overall survival.

4.4.1 Hormonal Therapy

Epidemiologic data on meningiomas is suggestive of a link between hormonal factors and development or progression of these tumors. The data has been controversial, with meningiomas being more frequent among women who had multiple pregnancies and among patients with history of breast cancer. However, early menarche and late menopause have not increased the risk of developing meningioma (Grunberg et al., 1991; Wen et al., 2010). Progesterone and androgen receptors are expressed on approximately two thirds of meningiomas and estrogen receptors are expressed on approximately 10% (Wen et al., 2009). Progesterone receptors are predominantly expressed in benign meningiomas with low proliferation indices and they are infrequently expressed in atypical and malignant meningiomas (Wolfsberger et al, 2004). Again, data for malignant meningiomas specifically is limited, likely due to their scarcity. Inhibition of sex hormone receptors has been tried in attempt to alter the course of recurrent meningioma, but without significant success.

4.4.1.1 Progesterone Receptor Inhibition

Progesterone receptor inhibition initially appeared promising, as several small studies showed some efficacy of anti-progestational drug *mifepristone.*

A group of 10 patients with 12 recurrent or primary inoperable meningiomas with recent evidence of tumor growth received 200 mg of mifepristone daily for 12 months (Lamberts et al., 1992). Progression of growth of 5 tumors in 4 patients, stable disease in 3 patients and regression of 4 tumors in 3 patients was shown on CT scan analysis. Five patients had subjective improvement in headache and general well-being. Mifepristone treatment resulted in control of tumor growth in 6 out of 10 patients. Three of them were noted to have tumor shrinkage.

Another study followed 14 patients with unresectable meningiomas treated with 200 mg of mifepristone daily for 2 to over 31 months (Grunberg et al., 1991). Five patients have shown signs of objective response, 3 have experienced subjective improvement.

These results prompted more comprehensive investigations. A phase III double-blind placebo-controlled randomized study analyzed data on 160 patients with unresectable non-malignant meningiomas, which have appeared or progressed within two years prior to enrollment (Grunberg et al., 2001). Patients were randomized to mifepristone and placebo group, 80 patients per arm. There was no significant difference in response: two mifepristone-treated patients and one placebo-treated patient had partial or unconfirmed responses.

A study following 28 patients with unresectable meningiomas treated with mifepristone for median duration of 35 months (Grunberg et al., 2006) has shown minor responses in 8 patients, 7 of whom were male or premenopausal female. The most common side effects were fatigue, hot flashes and gynecomastia/breast tenderness. Endometrial hyperplasia or polyps were noted in 3 patients and one patient developed peritoneal adenocarcinoma after 9 years of therapy.

Overall, the long-term administration of mifepristone appears to be clinically well tolerated, with modest effect on tumor control, better in subgroup of male and premenopausal female patients. Mifepristone's lack of efficacy may be explained in part by the loss of progesterone receptor expression in meningiomas with increased proliferation index and histologic grade. This is relevant because these advanced tumors are the type most likely to be enrolled into clinical studies (Grunberg et al., 2006; Wen et al., 2010).

4.4.1.2 Estrogen Receptor Inhibition

Estrogen receptor inhibition has been tried in a study on twenty-one patients with non-resectable refractory meningiomas (Goodwin et al., 1993). *Tamoxifen* 40 mg/m^2 was given BID for 4 days, then 10mg BID thereafter. Out of 19 patients that were eligible to continue the study, 1 achieved an MRI-documented partial response, while 2 had a minor CT-documented response of short duration (4 and 20 months). Six patients remained stable for a median duration of 31 months, while 10 (53%) demonstrated progression. This study, as well as the other rare reports fail to prove the benefits of estrogen receptor inhibition in treatment of meningiomas.

4.4.1.3 Androgen Receptor Inhibition

Androgen receptor inhibition with *flutamide* has been tried on a group of 6 patients with no response (Wen et al., 2010). There have been no published trials on androgen receptor antagonists in meningiomas.

4.4.2 Chemotherapy

As with other modalities of systemic treatment, chemotherapy has been mainly used for recurrent tumors after the surgical and radiation options have been exhausted. Available data comes from small clinical trials and case series. Further difficulty in interpreting the efficacy of chemotherapy is posed by the lack of data regarding the natural history of untreated meningiomas (Wen et al., 2010). Overall, most chemotherapeutics have only minimal activity against meningiomas.

4.4.2.1 Dacarbazine, Adriamycin, Ifosphamide and Mesna

Dacarbazine, adriamycin, ifosphamide and mesna were ineffective in treatment of meningiomas.

4.4.2.2 Combination of Cyclophosphamide, Adriamycin and Vincristine (CAV)

Combination of cyclophosphamide, adriamycin and vincristine (CAV) was studied on 14 patients with primary malignant meningiomas (Chamberlain, 1996). They all underwent surgery (gross-total in 4 and sub-total in 10), followed by radiotherapy. Two to four weeks after radiotherapy, all patients were treated with adjuvant chemotherapy that included CAV. Myelosuppression was the main serious adverse effect. Neuroradiographic response included 3 partial responses and 11 with stable disease. The median time to tumor progression was 4.6 years and median survival was 5.3 years. The conclusion was that the CAV therapy for malignant meningiomas is associated with acceptable toxicity and a modest improvement in survival when compared to patients treated with surgery alone.

4.4.2.3 Temozolomide (TMZ)

Temozolomide (TMZ) has been ineffective. A phase II study (Chamberlain et al., 2004) was conducted on 16 patients with refractory meningioma, previously treated with surgery and radiotherapy, but no prior chemotherapy. Temozolomide was administered orally for 42 consecutive days every 10 weeks. TMZ-related toxicity included anemia (25%), fatigue (18.7%), neutropenia (37.5%), seizures (6.3%) and thrombocytopenia (18.7%). None of the patients demonstrated a neuroradiographic complete or partial response.

4.4.2.4 Irinothecan

Irinothecan has shown inhibition of meningioma cell growth in vitro, but it was ineffective in vivo (Wen et al., 2010).

4.4.2.5 Hydroxyurea

Hydroxyurea, an oral ribonucleotide reductase inhibitor, arrests meningioma cell growth in the S phase of the cell cycle and induces apoptosis. Preliminary reports on use of hydroxyurea appeared promising, but the phase II studies that followed these initial results failed to prove significant efficacy. Many of the patients treated with hydroxyurea also received radiation therapy, making the interpretation of the results even more difficult (Wen et al., 2010). A phase II study of hydroxyurea for unresectable meningiomas (Swinnen et al., 2009) included patients with unresectable, measurable, residual or recurrent, histologically proven benign meningiomas. The study was closed after 29 patients were accrued, due to the slow subject recruitment rate. The objective response rate to chronic hydroxyurea therapy was estimated to ≤12%. Whether the stable disease rate seen differs in any way from what can be expected from the natural history of meningioma could not be determined from this phase II study design.

Another phase II study of hydroxyurea (Fuentes et al., 2004) included 43 patients presenting with unresectable meningioma with clinically and/or neuroradiologically documented progression. They received 20 mg/kg/day of hydroxyurea orally and were followed every 3 months with physical exam, MRI or CT imaging. Twenty-eight patients underwent surgery. Histology was benign in 18 and atypical in 10 patients. Objective response to hydroxyurea was found in only 3 patients (7%). Progressive disease was observed clinically or radiologically in 26 patients (60.5%). Of the eligible population (n=36 with clinically and/or radiologically proved progression of the disease at the time of entering the study), 2 achieved an objective response and 13 (36%) exhibited stabilization under hydroxyurea therapy, while 21 (58%) progressed under treatment. Overall tolerance of treatment was good, but anemia was observed in 28%, asthenia in 23.5% patients and skin toxicity in one patient. This study did not include any patients with known malignant meningiomas (WHO grade III).

4.4.2.6 Combinations of Hydroxyurea with Imatinib and with Verapamil

There are ongoing phase II clinical trials investigating *combinations of hydroxyurea* with *imatinib* and with *verapamil.*

4.4.3 Interferon α

Recombinant interferon alpha inhibits the growth of meningioma cells in vitro. There are several reports on small groups of patients (up to 12) showing resultant stable disease (Wen et al., 2010). A group of 6 patients with either a recurrent malignant meningioma or an unresectable meningioma was treated with interferon-α (Kaba et al., 1997). Two of the six meningiomas were regular, one was atypical and three were malignant. Five of six patients exhibited positive response to treatment, with stabilization of the size of the tumor in four patients and slight regression in one. The toxicity related to interferon was mild and well tolerated, mainly including flu-like symptoms in the beginning of therapy and pain at the injection site thereafter.

A phase II study of patients with recurrent, treatment-refractory, WHO grade I meningiomas (Chamberlain & Glantz, 2008) included 35 patients who all received prior surgery, radiotherapy and chemotherapy. On radiographic documentation of progressive disease, interferon-α was initiated at a dose of 10 million IU/m^2, subcutaneously every other day in 4-week long cycles. Concurrent dexamethsone was permitted for control of neurologic signs and symptoms. It was given orally to 12 patients. All the patients were followed with complete blood count, chemistry panel and MRI every 3 months. The main toxicities were fatigue, anemia and leucopenia, which required discontinuation in 3 patients and dose reduction in 7 patients. No patients demonstrated a neuroradiographic complete or partial response. Twenty-six patients demonstrated stable disease after the first 3 cycles of interferon, and 9 had progressive disease. The median time to tumor progression was 7 months. All but 3 patients died of disease progression. The median overall survival was 8 months (range 3-28 months). In contrast to previous small studies, this study was confined to patients who had histologcally documented WHO grade I meningiomas that had recurred despite undergoing 1 or more prior surgeries. In addition, all patients had failed external beam radiotherapy, half had received stereotactic radiotherapy, and nearly all (34 of 35 patients) had progressed despite previous chemotherapy. Malignant transformation to a higher grade meningioma may have occurred, and the results may be reflective of treating mixed grades of meningiomas. Interferon-α appears to have citostatic activity against heavily pretreated, recurrent meningiomas and could be considered as a palliative therapy for patients who have failed previous surgery and radiotherapy.

4.4.4 Somatostatin Analogs

Somatostatin receptors are expressed in nearly 90% of meningiomas (Norden et al., 2011; Wen et al., 2010).

4.4.4.1 Octreotide

There have been anecdotal reports of *octreotide* (long-acting somatostatin agonist) inhibiting growth in human meningiomas, but the small number of patients make the results difficult to interpret.

A report on three patients (Garcia-Luna et al., 1993) diagnosed with unresectable meningioma, which were treated with octreotide showed almost perfect tolerance to the drug. No change was observed by CT scan at the end of treatment course. The treatment was given for 6 to 16 weeks to each patient and the authors considered the short duration of the treatment to be a possible culprit in not seeing more favorable results.

A case report on a 54-year-old female with suspected pituitary adenoma (Jaffrain-Rea et al., 1998) has shown significant clinical and visual improvement during short-term octreotide therapy, contrasting with the lack of neuroradiological evidence of tumor shrinkage. The patient subsequently underwent transcranial surgery with a final diagnosis of meningioma.

In a study of 16 patients with recurrent meningiomas (Chamberlain et al., 2007) who had progressed radiographycally after prior surgery, radiotherapy and chemotherapy, presence of somatostatin receptors was confirmed using octreotide and SPECT scanning. Patients were prospectively treated with octreotide, 2-15 cycles on a monthly schedule, with minimal toxicity. The overall progression-free survival was 44% (7 patients) at 6 months. Thirty-one percent of patients demonstrated a partial radiographic response. Toxicity was minimal, suggesting that somatostatin analogues may offer novel, relatively non-toxic alternative treatment for recurrent meningiomas.

4.4.4.2 Pastreotide

Pastreotide is a long-acting somatostatin analog with a higher binding affinity for most somatostatin receptor subtypes than octreotide. In an open label, single arm phase II trial (Norden et al., 2011) pastreotide was given intramuscularly on monthly basis to patients with recurrent or progressive intracranial meningioma. Twenty-six participants have been accrued, 17 of whom (65%) have atypical/malignant meningiomas with previous radiation therapy. Twenty-two tumors show at least intermediate octreotide uptake. There are no radiographic responses. Of 22 evaluable patients, 16 (73%) achieved stable disease. Toxicity included hyperglycemia in 6 patients and elevated lipase in 2 patients. Pastreotide appears to be well tolerated somatostatin analog that is under investigation for heavily pre-treated recurrent meningiomas.

4.4.5 Molecularly Targeted Agents

An increased understanding of the cell signaling pathways has led to the identification of other potential targets for therapeutic intervention. Molecular drugs are designed to target the pathways involved in cell growth, proliferation and angiogenesis. Unlike gliomas, where the blood-brain barrier limits the penetration of many therapeutic agents, the penetration of targeted agents in meningiomas is unlikely to be a major issue (Wen et al.,

2010). As with the other therapies, data for molecularly targeted agents used on malignant meningiomas specifically is unavailable.

4.4.5.1 Platelet Derived Growth Factor (PDGF)

Platelet derived growth factor (PDGF) stimulates tumor cell growth in various tumors. PDGF receptors are expressed in most meningiomas. In a study of expression of PDGF and its receptor in 61 meningiomas by immunohistochemistry and in situ hybridization (Yang & Xu, 2001), it was found that almost all expressed PDGFBB and PDGFβ receptor and the positive rate of PDGFAA was 49%. Only 2 meningiomas expressed PDGFα receptor. The positive rate and immunostaining intensity of PDGFBB and PDGFβ receptor were higher in atypical meningiomas than in benign types. The proliferative activity was found to be higher in atypical meningiomas than in benign types, as evaluated by proliferating cell nuclear antigen labeling index (PCNA LI). The expression of PDGFBB and PDGFβ receptor was increasing with increase of PCNA LI. Therefore, the conclusion was that the overexpression of PDGFBB and PDGFβ receptor in meningiomas correlates with grade of meningiomas and the proliferative activity of meningiomas; PDGFBB/Rβ autocrine loop may play critical role in the pathogenesis of meningiomas.

Inhibition of PDGF receptors with *imatinib* was tried in a phase II study, which enrolled 23 patients with recurrent meningiomas (Wen et al., 2009). Out of 22 eligible patients, 13 had benign, 5 atypical and 5 malignant meningiomas. Imatinib was given at a dose of 600 mg/day for the first 4-week cycle, and then gradually increased to 800 mg/day for subsequent cycles. Tissue was available only from minority of patients, but in these specimens there was uniform distribution of PDGF receptors. Out of 19 patients evaluable for response, 10 had progression at first scan and 9 were stable. There were no complete or partial responses. For atypical and malignant meningiomas, median progression-free survival was 2 months. The study was closed due to slow subject accrual. It has shown that imatinib was well tolerated, but ineffective in treatment of recurrent meningiomas.

A recent in vitro trial on primary meningioma cells is suggesting synergistic activity of *imatinib* and protease inhibitor and pro-apoptotic agent *nelfinavir* (Gupta et al., 2007). Primary meningioma cells responded better to combination therapy than to imatinib alone. Combination was also more effective than imatinib alone on in vivo models. The investigation of this combination has still not reached clinical phase.

The combination of *imatinib* and *hydroxyurea* for treatment of recurrent meningioma has been tried in a phase II study at Duke University (Wen et al., 2010). The results are not available yet.

Several other PDGFR inhibitors are undergoing evaluation: *tandutinib, dasatinib, nilotinib, sunitinib, pazopanib* and *CHIR 265.* They are tried for variety of cancers, and some of them might be effective for treatment of meningiomas.

4.4.5.2 Epidermal Growth Factor Receptor (EGFR) Inhibitors and Antibodies

Epidermal growth factor receptor (EGFR) is overexpressed in over 60% of meningiomas (Johnson & Toms, 2005; Wen et al., 2010). EGF and transforming growth factor α (TGFα) activate these receptors stimulating meningioma cell proliferation in vitro (Johnson & Toms, 2005). Increased TGFα immunoreactivity in meningioma has been associated with aggressive growth. TGFα is also present in the surrounding cerebrospinal fluid. In contrast, one immunohistochemical study on 84 meningiomas (36 benign, 29 atypical and 19 malignant) suggested that atypical meningiomas without EGFR expression had a statistically worse prognosis compared to atypical EGFR-expressing tumors (Smith et al., 2007). The same tendency was not evident in cases of benign or malignant meningiomas. It is suspected that the atypical tumors lacking EGFR reactivity utilize potent alternative growth-stimulatory pathways.

EGFR inhibitors *erlotinib* and *gefitinib* were evaluated in an open label, single arm, phase II study for recurrent malignant meningiomas (Norden et al., 2010). Twenty-five eligible patients were enrolled. Sixteen (64%) of them received gefitinib and nine (36%) erlotinib. Eight patients (32%) had benign tumors, nine (36%) atypical and eight (32%) malignant. There were no objective imaging responses, but 8 patients (32%) maintained stable disease. Although treatment was well tolerated, neither gefitinib nor erlotinib appear to have significant activity against recurrent meningioma.

In addition to gefitinib and erlotinib, there is a number of other EGFR inhibitors currently undergoing evaluations (*lapatinib, neratinib, BIBW2992, PF00299804, ZD6474*). These inhibit EGFR more effectively or inhibit other tyrosine kinases also, potentially increasing their therapeutic benefit (Wen et al., 2010).

EGFR monoclonal antibodies have been effective for some systemic malignancies, but they have not been generally used for brain tumors because of the concern regarding the ability to cross blood-brain barrier in sufficient concentration. However, crossing the blood-brain barrier is not a factor in most meningiomas, so it is possible that these antibodies may be effective in these tumors (Wen et al., 2010).

4.4.5.3 Angiogenesis Inhibitors

Inhibition of angiogenesis has been an increasingly important approach to treating various cancers. Meningiomas are highly vascular tumors that derive their blood supply predominantly from meningeal vessels supplied by external carotid artery, with additional supply from cerebral pial vessels (Wen et al., 2010). Data on angiogenesis inhibition in treatment of meningioma is very limited. Vascular endothelial growth factor (VEGF) plays a central role in tumor angiogenesis. Anti-VEGF monoclonal antibody *bevacizumab* has significantly improved outcome in several systemic malignancies as well as in glioblastoma. At least one case report described a partial response in a patient with a progressing anaplastic meningioma (Puchner et al., 2010). Inhibitors of VEGF receptors, such as *sorafenib* and *sunitinib* have prolonged survival in renal cell carcinoma and GIST. Expression of VEGF and VEGFR on meningiomas increases with tumor grade (10-fold in malignant meningioma as compared to benign) (Lamszus et al., 2000). VEGF also plays an important role in the formation of peritumoral edema, which adds to the morbidity of these tumors (Provias et al., 1997). Inhibitors of VEGF and VEGFR have the potential to inhibit angiogenesis, as well as to decrease peritumoral edema.

5. Prognosis

WHO grade III tumors, including malignant meningiomas, are significantly more likely to be invasive and have a local recurrence following the initial treatment (even gross total resection). Prognosis worsens with the more poor differentiation of the tumors (Palma et al., 1997; Park & McLaren, 2009; Pasquier et al., 2008). High mitotic rate is a significant prognostic factor, as well as the poor Karnofski performance status (Pasquier et al., 2008). This leads to overall shorter survival as compared to patients with WHO grade I and II tumors. Several trials have elucidated this observation.

In a study of 1098 surgically treated patients (Yang et al., 2008), 40 were classified as atypical and 24 as anaplastic. 10-year survival and recurrence-free survival rates for patients with atypical tumors (WHO grade II) were 90 and 87%, respectively. In contrast, the patients with anaplastic (WHO grade III), 3 and 5-year recurrence-free survival rates were 50 and 29%, respectively.

Prognosis is also worse for partially resected tumors as compared to completely resected ones. However, the most available data was collected prior to development of adjuvant therapies, which do improve prognosis.

Simpson grade I resection can be reliably performed on convexity meningiomas and regardless of malignant histological findings, it can improve prognosis (Wen et al., 2010).

To better understand the prognostic differences between atypical and malignant meningiomas and the influence of extent of surgical excision on post-operative course, 42 cases of atypical and 29 of malignant meningiomas were studied (Palma et al., 1997). Survival at 5 and 10 years was 95% and 79%, respectively in patients with atypical meningiomas. It was 64.3% and 34.5% in patients with malignant meningiomas. Recurrence-free survival and median time to recurrence were also significantly longer in patients with atypical meningiomas than in patients with malignant tumors: 11.9 versus 2 years and 5 versus 2 years, respectively. Six (26%) of the atypical meningiomas became malignant. Simpson grade I resection and location in the cerebral convexity, which were closely related, were found to be associated with a significantly better clinical course in the entire series. Patients with atypical meningiomas fared better than those with malignant meningiomas after incomplete surgical resection, but the difference was not statistically significant. This study has shown that radical extirpation and histological findings were significantly related to prolonged survival.

Another study on 13 patients with grade III meningiomas (as defined by WHO 2007 classification), evaluated their outcomes (Rosenberg et al., 2009). A total of 24 surgeries were performed, including 13 primary, 7 salvage and 4 second salvage. Also, 14 courses of radiotherapy were administered. A trend was seen toward longer survival for patients who had received adjuvant radiotherapy after initial surgery as compared to those treated with surgery alone. This study confirmed the older observations of generally poor outcomes for malignant meningiomas and the tendency for extended survival in patients receiving adjuvant radiotherapy in comparison to those treated only surgically.

Hisopathological characteristics of tumors have a leading role in bringing the prognosis. It is important to keep in mind that tumors that were embolized prior to resection can change their microscopic appearance making histological analysis more difficult (Matsuda et al., 2011; see 4.1).

6. Conclusion

Malignant meningiomas display a tendency for post-surgical recurrence, which significantly increases for multicentric and recurrent disease. Compared to benign meningiomas, malignant meningiomas also display a shorter interval to recurrence. The information on malignant meningiomas as an entity separate from their benign and atypical counterparts is scarce, due to their rare occurrence. Furthermore, the classification of tumors has changed over the years, making it more difficult to compare the older observations with the new ones. There are no randomized prospective trials evaluating any aspect of management of these tumors.

However, from all the available data some general conclusions can be made. The patients who undergo complete surgical resection tend to have longer survival than those with partial resection. Pre-operative embolization, when feasible, can be helpful in achieving better surgical results. Adjuvant radiotherapy has shown significant benefits when it comes to progression-free survival rates and overall survival. In unresectable tumors, radiation alone can be helpful as well. Systemic therapy, including hormonal, chemotherapy, interferon and somatostatin analogs, has for the most part failed to show much benefit. The molecularly targeted agents have shown efficacy in tumors requiring systemic treatment. Further investigations on malignant meningiomas is warranted in order to improve the current treatment practices and ultimately ameliorate the prognosis for patients affected by these rare tumors.

7. Acknowledgement

We would like to thank our medical student Khurram Tariq for his kind help with this chapter.

8. References

Aiyama H, Nakai K, Yamamoto T, Narai T, Kumada H, Ishikawa E, Isobe T, Endo K, Takada T, Yoshida F, Shibata Y & Matsumura A (2011). *A Clinical Trial Protocol for Second Line Treatment of Malignant Brain Tumors with BNCT at University of Tskuba,* Appl Radiat Isot. 2011 Jul 19. (Epub ahead of print)

Blitshteyn S, Crook JE & Jaeckle KA (2008). *Is There an Association Between Meningioma and Hormone Replacement Therapy?,* J Clin Oncol. 2008; 26(2): 279

Borovich B & Doron Y (1986). *Recurrence of Intracranial Meningiomas: The Role Played by Regional Multicentricity,* J Neurosurg. 1986 Jan; 64(1): 58-63

Borovich B, Doron Y, Braun J, Guilburd JN, Zaaroor M, Goldsher D, Lemberger A, Gruszkiewicz J & Feinsod M (1986). *Recurrence of Intracranial Meningiomas: The Role Played by Regional Multicentricity. Part 2: Clinical and Radiological Aspects,* J Neurosurg. 1986 Aug; 65(2): 168-71

Carli DF, Sluzewski M, Beute GN & van Rooij WJ (2010). *Complications of Particle Embolization of Meningiomas: Frequency, Risk Factors and Outcome,* AJNR Am J Neuroradiol. 2010 Jan; 31(1): 152-4. Epub 2009 Sep 3

CBTRUS (2011). http://www.cbtrus.org/2007-2008/2007-20081.html (accessed on 10 Aug 2011)

Chamberlain MC (1996). *Adjuvant Combined Modality Therapy for Malignant Meningiomas,* J Neurosurg. 1996; 84(5): 733

Chamberlain MC, Tsao-Wei DD & Groshen S (2004). *Temozolamide for Treatment-Resistant Recurrent Meningioma,* Neurology, 2004; 62(7): 1210

Chamberlain MC, Glantz MJ & Fadul CE (2007). *Recurrent Meningioma: Salvage Therapy With Long-Acting Somatostatin Analogue,* Neurology, 2007; 69(10): 969

Chamberlain MC & Glantz MJ (2008). *Interferon-Alpha For Recurrent World Health Organization Grade I Intracranial Meningiomas,* Cancer, 2008; 113(8): 2146

Di Chiro G, Hatazawa J, Katz DA, Rizzoli HV & De Michele DJ (1987). *Glucose Utilization by Intracranial Meningiomas as an Index of Tumor Aggressivity and Probability of Recurrence: A PET Study,* Radiology. 1987 Aug; 164(2): 521-6

Dziuk TW, Woo S, Butler EB, Thornby J, Grossman R, Dennis WS, Lu H, Carpenter LS & Chiu JK (1998). *Malignant Meningioma: An Indication for Initial Aggressive Surgery and Adjuvant Radiotherapy,* Journal of Neuro-Oncology 37: 177-188, 1998

Fuentes S, Chinot O, Dufour H, Paz-Paredes A, Métellus P, Barrie-Attarian M & Grisoli F (2004). *Hydroxyurea Treatment for Unresectable Meningioma,* Neurochirurgie, 2004 Sep; 50(4): 461-7

Garcia-Luna PP, Relimpio F, Pumar A, Pereira JL, Leal-Cerro A, Trujillo F, Cortés A & Astorga R (1993). *Clinical Use of Octreotide In Unresectable Meningiomas. A Report of Three Cases,* J Neurosurg Sci. 1993; 37(4): 237

Goodwin JW, Crowley J, Eyre HJ, Stafford B, Jaeckle KA & Towsend JJ (1993). *A Phase II Evaluation of Tamoxifen in Unresectable or Refractory Meningiomas: A Southwest Oncology Group Study,* J Neurooncol. 1993; 15(1): 75

Goldsmith BJ, Wara WM, Wilson CB & Larson DA (1994). *Postoperative Irradiation for Subtotally Resected Meningiomas. A Retrospective Analysis of 140 Patients Treated from 1967 to 1990,* J Neurosurg. 1994 Feb; 80(2): 195-201

Grossman, RI & Yousem DM (2003), Neoplasm of the Brain, in *Neuroradiology: The Requisites,* Thrall JH, pp 97-105, Mosby, ISBN-13: 978-0-323-00508-1, ISBN-10: 0-323-00508-X, USA

Grunberg SM, Weiss MH, Spitz IM, Ahmadi J, Sadun A, Russell CA, Lucci L & Stevenson LL (1991). *Treatment of Unresectable Meningiomas with the Antiprogesterone Agent Mifepristone,* J Neurosurg. 1991 Jun; 74(6): 861-6.

Grunberg SM, Weiss MH, Russell CA, Spitz IM, Ahmadi J, Sadun A, Sitruk-Ware R (2006). *Long-Term Administration of Mifepristone (RU486): Clinical Tolerance During Extended Treatment of Meningioma,* Cancer Invest. 2006 Dec; 24(8): 727-33.

Grunberg SM, Rankin C, Townsend J, Ahmadi J, Feun L, Fredericks R, Russell C, Kabbinavar F, Barger GR & Stelzer KJ (2001). *Phase III Double-Blind Randomized Placebo-Controlled Study of Mifepristone (RU) for the Treatment of Unresectable Meningioma,* Proc Am Soc Clin Oncol 20: 2001 (abstr 222)

Gupta V, Samuleson CG, Su S & Chen TC (2007). *Nelfinavir Potentiation of Imatinib Cytotoxicity in Meningioma Cells via Survivin Inhibition,* Neurosurg Focus. 2007;23(4):E9

Hanft S, Canoll P & Bruce JN (2010). *A Review of Malignant Meningiomas: Diagnosis, Characteristics and Treatment,* J Neurooncol (2010) 99: 433-443

Hsu CC, Pai CY, Kao HW, Hsueh CJ, Hsu WL & Lo CP (2010). *Do Aggressive Imaging Features Correlate with Advanced Histopathological Grade in Meningiomas?,* J Clin Neurosci. 2010; 17(5): 584

Jääskeläinen J, Haltia M & Servo A (1986). *Atypical and Anaplastic Meningiomas: Radiology, Surgery, Radiotherapy and Outcome,* Surg Neurol. 1986 Mar; 25(3): 233-42

Jaffrain-Rea ML, Minniti G, Santoro A, Bastianello S, Tamburrano G, Gulino A & Cantore G (1998). *Visual Improvement During Octreotide Therapy in a Case of Episellar Meningioma,* Clin Neurol Neurosurg. 1998; 100(1): 40

Jhawar BS, Fuchs CS, Colditz GA & Stampfer MJ (2003). *Sex Steroid Hormone Exposures and Risk for Meningioma,* J neurosurg. 2003; 99(5): 848

Johnson M & Toms S (2005). *Mitogenic Signal Transduction Pathways in Meningiomas: Novel Targets for Meningioma Chemotherapy?,* J Neuropathol Exp Neurol. 2005 Dec; 64(12):1029-36

Kaba SE, DeMonte F, Bruner JM, Kyritsis AP, Jaeckle KA, Levin V & Young WKA (1997). *The Treatment of Recurrent Unresectable And Malignant Meningiomas With Interferon Alpha-2B,* Neurosurgery, 1997; 40(2): 271

Kallio M, Sankila R, Hakulinen T & Jääskeläinen J (1992). *Factors Affecting Operative and Excess LongTerm Mortality in 935 Patients with Intracranial Meningioma,* Neurosurgery: July 1992 - Volume 31 - Issue 1 - p 2-12

Lamberts SW, Tanghe HL, Avezaat CJ, Braakman R, Wijngaarde R, Koper JW & de Jong H (1992). *Mifepristone (RU 486) Treatment of Meningiomas,* J Neurol Neurosurg Psychiatry. 1992 June; 55(6): 486–490

Lamszus K, Lengler U, Schmidt NO, Stavrou D, Ergün S & Westphal M (2000). *Vascular Endothelial Growth Factor, Hepatocyte Growth Factor/Scatter Factor, Basic Fibroblast Growth Factor, and Placenta Growth Factor in Human Meningiomas and Their Relation to Angiogenesis and Malignancy,* Neurosurgery. 2000 Apr;46(4):938-47; discussion 947-8

Marosi C, Hassler M, Roessler K, Reni M, Sant M, Mazza E & Vecht C (2008). *Meningioma,* Crit Rev Oncol Hematol. 2008; 67(2): 153

Matsuda K, Takeuchi H, Arai Y, Kitai R, Hosoda T, Tsunetoshi K, Arishima H, Sato K & Kikuta K (2011). *Atypical and Ischemic Features of Embolized Meningiomas,* Brain Tumor Pathol DOI 10.1007/s10014-011-0058-9

Mastronardi L, Ferrante L, Qasho R, Ferrari V, Tatarelli R & Fortuna A (1995). *Intracranial Meningiomas in the 9th Decade of Life: A Retrospective Study of 17 Surgical Cases,* Neurosurgery. 1995 Feb; 36(2): 270-4.

Maxwell M, Shih SD, Galanopoulos T, Hedley-Whyte ET & Cosgrove GR (1998). *Familial Meningioma: Analysis of Expression of Neurofibromatosis 2 Protein Merlin. Report of Two Cases,* J Neurosurg. 1998; 88(3): 562

Mendenhall WM, Morris CG, Amdur RJ, Foote KD & Friedman WA (2003). *Radiotherapy alone or after subtotal resection for benign skull base meningiomas,* Cancer. 2003 Oct 1; 98(7): 1473-82

National Comprehensive Cancer Network® (NCCN) (2011). *NCCN Guidelines™ Version 2.2011 Central Nervous System Cancers, MENI-1,* http://www.nccn.org/professionals/physician_gls/f_guidelines.asp#site

Neglia JP, Robison LL, Stovall M, Liu Y, Packer RJ, Hammond S, Yasui Y, Kasper CE, Mertens AC, Donaldson SS, Meadows AT, Inskip PD (2006). *New Primary Neoplasms of the Central Nervous System in Survivors of Childhood Cancer:Aa Report from the Childhood Cancer Survivor Study,* J Natl Cancer Inst. 2006 Nov 1; 98(21): 1528-37

Norden AD, Raizer JJ, Abrey LE, Lamborn KR, Lassman AB, Chang SM, Yung WK, Gilbert MR, Fine HA, Mehta M, Deangelis LM, Cloughesy TF, Robins HI, Aldape K,

Dancey J, Prados MD, Lieberman F & Wen PY (2010). *Phase II Trials of Erlotinib or Gefitinib in Patients With Recurrent Meningioma,* J Neurooncol. 2010; 96(2): 211

Norden AD, Hammond S, Drappatz J, Phuphanich S, Reardon DA, Wong E, Plotkin SR, Lesser GJ, Raizer JJ, Batchelor T, Quant EC, Beroukhim R, Kaley TJ, Muzikansky A, Ciampa AS, Doherty LM, Smith KH, Gerard M, Sceppa C & Wen PY (2011). *Phase II Study of Monthly Pasireotide LAR (SOM230C) for Recurrent or Progressive Meningioma,* J Clin Oncol 29: 2011 ASCO Annual Meeting, abstract No 2040

Oka H, Kurata A, Kawano N, Saegusa H, Kobayashi I, Ohmomo T, Miyasaka Y & Fujii K. (1998) *Preoperative Superselective Embolization of Skull-Base Meningiomas: Indications and Limitations,* J Neurooncol. 1998 Oct; 40(1): 67-71

Palma L, Celli P, Franco C, Cervoni L & Cantore G (1997). *Long-Term Prognosis for Atypical and Malignant Meningiomas: A study of 71 Surgical Cases,* J Neurosurg. 1997; 86(5): 793

Park JK & McLaren Black P (2009). *Biology and Clinical Features of Meningioma,* www.uptodate.com, October 21, 2009

Park JK, McLaren Black P & Shih H (2010b). *Treatment of Meningiomas,* www.uptodate.com, January 12, 2010

Park JK, McLaren Black P & Wrensch (2010a). *Meningioma: Epidemiology, Risk Factors and Pathology,* www.uptodate.com, November 18, 2010

Pasquier D, Bijmolt S, Veninga T, Rezvoy N, Villa S, Krengli M, Weber DC, Baumert BG, Canyilmaz E, Yalman D, Szutowicz E, Tzuk-Shina T & Mirimanoff RO (2008). *Atypical and Malignant Meningioma: Outcome and Prognostic Factors in 119 Irradiated Patients. A multicenter, Retrospective Study of the Rare Cancer Network,* Int J Radiat Oncol Biol Phys. 2008 Aug 1; 71(5): 1388-93. Epub 2008 Mar 4

Perry A, Scheithauer BW, Stafford SL, Lohse CM & Wollan PC (1999). *"Malignancy" in Meningiomas: A Clinicopathologic Study of 116 Patients, with Grading Implications,* Cancer. 1999; 85(9): 2046

Preston-Martin S, Paganini-Hill A, Henderson BE, Pike MC & Wood C (1980). *Case-Control Study of Intracranial Meningiomas in Women in Los Angeles County, California,* J Natl Cancer Inst. 1980; 65(1): 67

Preston-Martin S, Pogoda JM, Schlehofer B, Blettner M, Howe GR, Ryan P, Menegoz F, Giles GG, Rodvall Y, Choi NW, Little J & Arslan A (1998). *An International Case-Control Study of Adult Glioma and Meningioma: The Role of Head Trauma.* Int J Epidemiol. 1998; 27(4): 579

Provias J, Claffey K, delAguila L, Lau N, Feldkamp M & Guha A, Meningiomas (1997). *Role of Vascular Endothelial Growth Factor/Vascular Permeability Factor in Angiogenesis and Peritumoral Edema,* Neurosurgery: May 1997 - Volume 40 - Issue 5 - pp 1016-102

Puchner MJA, Hans VH, Haratl A, Lohmann F, Glas M & Herrlinger U (2010), *Bevacizumab-Induced Regression of Anaplastic Meningioma,* Annals of Oncology, 2010 Dec; Vol 21, Issue 12, pp 2445-2446

Ron E, Modan B, Boice JD Jr, Alfandary E, Stovall M, Chetrit A & Katz L (1988). *Tumors of the Brain and Nervous System After Radiotherapy in Childhood,* N Engl J Med. 1988; 319(16): 1033

Rosen CL, Ammerman JM, Sekhar LN & Bank WO (2002). *Outcome Analysis of Preoperative Embolization in Cranial Base Surgery*, Acta Neurochir (Wien). 2002 Nov; 144(11): 1157-64

Rosenberg LA, Prayson RA, Lee J, Reddy C, Chao ST, Barnett GH, Vogelbaum MA & Suh JH (2009). *Long-Term Experience with Worls Health Organization Grade III (Malignant) Meningiomas at a Single Institution*, Int J Radiat Oncol Biol Phys. 2009; 74(2): 427

Salazar OM (1988). *Ensuring Local Control in Meningiomas*, Int J Radiat Oncol Biol Phys. 1988 Aug; 15(2): 501-4

Sawaya R, Zuccarello M, Elkalliny M & Nishiyama H (1992). *Postoperative Venous Thromboembolism and Brain Tumors: Part I. Clinical Profile*, J Neurooncol. 1992 Oct; 14(2): 119-25

Sawaya R & Glas-Greenwalt P (1992). *Postoperative Venous Thromboembolism and Brain Tumors: Part II. Hemostatic Profile*, J Neurooncol. 1992 Oct; 14(2): 127-34

Shapir J, Coblentz C, Malanson D, Ethier R & Robitaille Y (1985). *New CT Finding in Aggressive Meningioma*, AJNR Am J Neuroradiol. 1985 Jan-Feb; 6(1): 101-2

Simpson, D (1957). *The Recurrence of Intracranial Meningioma After Surgical Treatment*, J. Neurol. Neurosurg. Psychiat., 1957, 20, 22

Smith JS, Lal A, Harmon-Smith M, Bollen AW & McDermott MW (2007). *Association Between Absence of Epidermal Growth Factor Receptor Immunoreactivity and Poor Prognosis in Patients with Atypical Meningioma*, J Neurosurg. 2007 Jun; 106(6):1034-40

Sughrue ME, Sanai N, Shangari G, Parsa AT, Berger MS & McDermott MW (2010). *Outcome and Survival Following Primary and Repeat Surgery for World Health Organization Grade III Meningiomas*, J Neurosurg. 2010 Aug; 113(2): 202-9.

Swinnen LJ, Rankin C, Rushing EJ, Laura HF, Damek DM & Barger GR (2009). *Phase II Study of Hydroxyurea for Unresectable Meningioma (Southwest Oncology Group S9811)*, Journal of Clinical Oncology 2009, Vol 27, No 15S

Wen PY, Quant E, Drappatz J, Beroukhim R & Norden AD (2010). *Medical Therapies for Meningiomas*, J Neurooncol, 2010; 99(3): 365-378

Wen PY, Yung WK, Lamborn KR, Norden AD, Cloughesy TF, Abrey LE, Fine HA, Chang SM, Robins HI, Fink K, Deangelis LM, Mehta M, Di Tomaso E, Drappatz J, Kesari S, Ligon KL, Aldape K, Jain RK, Stiles CD, Egorin MJ & Prados MD (2009). *Phase II Study of Imatinib Mesylate for Recurrent Meningiomas (North American Brain Tumor Consortium Study 01-08)*, Neuro Oncol. 2009; 11(6): 853

WHO Classification of Tumors of the Central Nervous System (2007), Louis DN, Ohgaki, H, Wiestler OD & Cavenee WK, ISBN978-92-832-2430-2, Lyon (France)

Wigertz A, Lönn S, Mathiesen T, Ahlbom A, Hall P & Feychting M (2006). *Risk of Brain Tumors Associated with Exposure to Exogenous Female Sex Hormones*, Am J Epidemiol. 2006; 164(7): 629

Wolfsberger S, Doostkam S, Boecher-Schwarz HG, Roessler K, van Trotsenburg M, Hainfellner JA & Knosp E (2004). *Progesterone-Receptor Index in Meningiomas: Correlation with Clinico-Pathological Parameters and Review of the Literature*, Neurosurg Rev. 2004 Oct; 27(4): 238-45. Epub 2004 May 27

World Health Organization Classification of Tumors (WHO OMS), International Agency for Research on Cancer (IARC) (2000), Meningeal Tumors, in *Pathology and Genetics of*

Tumors of The Nervous System, Kleihues P & Cavenee WK, pp 175-184, IARC Press, ISBN 92 832 2409 4, Lyon (France)

Yang SY, Park CK, Park SH, Kim DG, Chung YS & Jung HW (2008). *Atypical and Anaplastic Meningiomas: Prognostic Implications of Clinicopathological Features,* J Neurol Neurosurg Psychiatry. 2008 May; 79(5): 574-80. Epub 2007 Aug 31

Yang SY & Xu GM (2001). *Expression of PDGF and Its Receptor as well as Their Relationship to Proliferating Activity and Apoptosis of Meningiomas in Human Meningiomas,* J Clin Neurosci. 2001 May; 8 Suppl 1:49-53.

2

Management of Lumbar Spinal Meningioma: A Systematic Review

Hiroki Hirabayashi
Department of Orthopaedic Surgery, Shinshu University School of Medicine
Japan

1. Introduction

Meningiomas are typically benign, slowly growing tumors. Meningiomas of the spine are most commonly intradural, extramedullary lesions and account of 25% - 46% of all spinal cord tumors in adults (Peker et al., 2005). Approximately 80% of spinal meningiomas occur in the thoracic spine, followed in frequency by cervical and lumbar lesions (Helseth et al., 1989; Levy et al., 1982; Roux et al., 1996; Solero et al., 1989) and little is known about lumbar spinal meningiomas. In this chapter, the outcomes of clinical studies regarding treatment of lumbar spinal meningioma are reviewed.

2. Systemic reviewing

A literature review regarding surgical treatment and clinical outcome of lumbar spinal meningioma was performed.

2.1 Search strategy

A MEDLINE database search was performed with the key words "spinal meningioma" and "lumbar." The key word "spinal meningioma" was only searched in combination. The limits included "English" for the language category, "humans" for the study category, and "added to MEDLINE in the last 10 years" for the period of publication. The date of the latest search was December 2010.

2.2 Selection criteria

Clinical papers concerning the surgical management of lumbar and lumbosacral spinal meningiomas that included treatment options and outcome analysis on follow-up were eligible for evaluation. Reference lists in articles were examined for further pertinent material. Articles were included when they contained quantitative data about the outcome and recurrence rate after surgical treatment of spinal meningiomas.

2.3 Selection and analysis of articles

Information extracted from eligible studies included the following variables: study design, patient age, gender, instrumentation, histological features, functional outcome, recurrence rate, and adjuvant therapies.

2.4 Baseline data

The MEDLINE review yielded one case series (Voulgaris et al, 2010) and nine case reports (Boet et al., 2004; Chen et al., 2004; Colen et al., 2009; Conrad et al., 2001; Epstein et al., 2005; Hirabayashi et al., 2009; Lee et al., 2002; Mizutani et al., 2002; Oviedo et al., 2005) involving 10 patients with lumbar and lumbosacral spinal meningiomas. The design was retrospective in all ten studies. Information about the age, gender, surgical approach, histological features, surgical outcome on long-term follow-up, recurrence rates, and adjuvant therapies are listed in Table 1.

Author Year	Age	Sex	Symptom	Surgical Approach	Histology	Surgical Outcome
Conrad 2001	31	F	Lumbosacral pain	Posterior	Metastatic meningioma	NA
Lee 2002	51	F	Low back pain and sciatica	Posterior - anterior - posterior	Metastatic meningioma	Significant improvement
Mizutani 2002	20	F	Low back pain and numbness	Posterior	Transitional meningioma	Significant improvement
Boet 2004	34	M	Low back pain and leg pain	Posterior	Clear cell meningioma	Significant improvement
Chen 2004	41	F	Sciatica	Posterior	Clear cell meningioma	Significant improvement
Epstein 2005	41	F	Progressive paraparesis	Posterior	Clear cell meningioma	Significant improvement
Oviedo 2005	7	M	Sciatica	NA	Clear cell meningioma	NA
Colen 2009	13	F	Low back pain and leg pain	Posterior	Clear cell meningioma	NA
Hirabayashi 2009	82	F	Leg pain	Posterior	Metaplastic meningioma	Significant improvement
Voulgaris 2010	63	F	Motor deficits	posterior	Psammomatous meningioma	NA

F: Female, M: Male, NA: not available

Table 1. Literature review of studies on lumbar spinal meningioma

Author Year	Complication	Tumor Recurrence	Adjuvant Treatment	Comment
Conrad 2001	No	Yes	Radiotherapy	Malignant meningioma
Lee 2002	No	Yes	Radiotherapy	Meningothelious meningioma
Mizutani 2002	No	No	No	Possibly induced by sex steroid pills
Boet 2004	No	No	Radiotherapy	
Chen 2004	No	No	NA	Renal transplant recipient
Epstein 2005	No	No	No	
Oviedo 2005	NA	No	No	
Colen 2009	NA	No	Radiotherapy	
Hirabayashi 2009	No	No	No	Without dural reconstruction
Voulgaris 2010	No	No	NA	

NA: not available

Table 1. (continued) Literature review of studies on lumbar spinal meningioma

2.5 Patient characteristics

The average age was 38.3 years (range, 7 - 82 years). There were two males and eight females. Patients' symptoms until surgery were low back pain and leg pain (sciatica) in 4 patients, leg pain (sciatica) in 3, neurological deficit in 2, and lumbosacral pain in 1. One patient was a very rare case of orally ingested sex hormone pills inducing meningioma (Mizutani et al., 2002), and another patient was also a rare case because she was a renal transplant recipient (Chen et al., 2004).

2.6 Surgical approach and outcome

All of the surgeries were performed via the posterior approach except in 1 case (Lee at al., 2002), in which the meningioma was present at the lumbosacral spine and was resected via the posterior-anterior-posterior approach. All cases showed significant improvement and benefit from surgery.

2.7 Tumor histology

The most common tumor histology was clear cell meningioma (5 patients), followed by metastatic meningioma (2), metaplastic meningioma (1), psammomatous meningioma (1), and transitional meningioma (1). In patients with metastatic lumbar spinal meningioma, the tumor histology was malignant meningioma and meningotheliomatous meningioma, which was similar to that of the primary intracranial tumor in one case each.

2.8 Complications and recurrence rates

There were no incidences of intraoperative mortality or morbidity. Tumor recurrence occurred in 2 patients, in both of whom the tumor histology was metastatic meningioma.

2.9 Adjuvant treatment

Postoperative adjuvant radiotherapy was administered in 4 of 8 patients (50%). Adjuvant chemotherapy was not provided in any patients.

3. Clinics

Spinal meningiomas are usually benign, slow-growing tumors with a long clinical history until a diagnosis is made. The most common location of spinal meningiomas is the thoracic spine. The percentage of thoracic spinal meningiomas in the literature review ranged from 64% to 84%, that of cervical meningiomas from 14% to 27%, and that of lumbar meningiomas from 2% to 14% (Gezen et al., 2000; Gottfried et al., 2003; King et al., 1998; Klekamp et al., 1999; Levy et al., 1982; Namer et al., 1987; Peker et al., 2005; Roux et al., 1996; Solero et al., 1989). Clinical symptoms are typically dependent on the tumor location with respect to the spinal cord or nerve roots, the rate of tumor growth, and the extent of spinal cord and/or cauda equina compression. The most common presenting symptom in this series was low back pain and leg pain (sciatica), followed by leg pain (sciatica), neurological deficit, and lumbosacral pain. The pain is often constant, and may be described as burning or aching in quality. Pain and motor patterns may obscure a systematic clinical presentation in these patients as high cervical lesions may present as occipital headache (McCormick et al., 1990), syringomyelia, and Brown-Séquard syndrome (Parsa et al., 2004), whereas thoracic neoplasms may be disguised as visceral pathology (McCormick et al., 1990). Less commonly, motor weakness, spasticity, sensory loss (hypoesthesia, paresthesia, or anesthesia), numbness, ataxic gait, or bowel and bladder dysfunction may be the initial presentation that arouses clinical attention (Gezen et al., 2000; King et al., 1998; Klekamp et al., 1999; Traul et al., 2007; Van Goethem et al., 2004). In this series, however, numbness and/or neurological deficits were frequent symptoms in patients with lumbar spinal meningioma.

4. Epidemiology

Spinal meningiomas may affect people of all ages, but they are most commonly seen among individuals between the fifth and seventh decades of life (Albanese et al., 2002; Solero et al., 1989; Tredway et al., 2006; Traul et al., 2007). In the World Health Organization (WHO) histological classification of meningiomas, the majority of cases correspond to WHO grade I (benign biotypes). However, rare histological variants, *i.e.,* clear cell and choroid meningioma (WHO grade II) and anaplastic meningioma (WHO grade III), are predictors of significant risk of local recurrence, aggressive biological behavior, and ominous prognosis. The most prognostic variables for refractory clinical behavior are histological grade and extent of tumor resection (Caroli et al., 2004). These tumors account for 25% - 46% of all primary intraspinal neoplasms (Peker et al., 2005). Women disproportionately (70%) harbor the intradural varieties, whereas there is a male predisposition in a small subset of spinal lesions (McCormick et al., 1990; Solero et al., 1989; Traul et al., 2007). Spinal meningiomas occur with highest frequency (80%) in the posterior, posterolateral or lateral thoracic region, followed by the anterior cervical region (15%), and infrequently in the lumbosacral region (5%) in women (Gottfried et al., 2003; McCormick et al., 1990). However, 50% of spinal meningiomas occur in the thoracic region and 40% in the cervical region in men (Van Goethem et al., 2004). Meningiomas show a greater predominance in the upper cervical region and foramen magnum than other tumors (McCormick et al., 1990). Due to their ventral or ventrolateral predisposition within the upper cervical region, spinal meningiomas may encase or surround the vertebral artery, but rarely infiltrate (Parsa et al., 2004). In the present series, most lumbar spinal meningiomas occurred in the third or fourth decade, and there was a significant difference in age between patients with clear cell meningiomas and those with another meningiomas, with the former occurring more often in younger patients. In contrast to other intradural tumors, there is a strong female predominance with a female/male ratio of 3:1 to 4:1 among patients with spinal meningiomas (Gezen et al., 2000; Gottfried et al., 2003). The female/male ratio in the present series was similar to those in previous reports.

5. Imaging

The current standard diagnostic method for spinal tumors is magnetic resonance imaging (MRI). MRI provides precise information about tumor localization (affected segment, relation to spinal cord and nerve root, and relation of the tumor to the dura), the extent of spinal cord compression, and further information about the spinal cord and the tumor itself; the presence of cord edema and intratumoral signal changes such as necrosis, hematoma, or calcification (Schroth et al., 1987). Spinal meningiomas are usually isointense to the spinal cord (T1- and T2-weighted MRI) and show enhancement after administration of contrast medium (Gd). There have been suggestions regarding the differentiation of one clinical entity from another (dural tail, broad dural contrast of meningioma, more lateral position of schwannomas, and relation to the nerve root); however, in this series, reliable differentiation between lumbar spinal clear cell meningiomas and other tumors (renal metastasis, ependymoma, neurilemmoma, and neurofibroma) by MRI was not possible (Chen et al., 2004; Epstein et al., 2005).

6. Diagnosis

The most frequent histological types among the Grade I tumors in our and the published series were the meningothelial and psammomatous types (Gezen et al., 2000; Gottfried et al., 2003; King et al., 1998; Klekamp et al., 1993; Levy et al., 1982; Namer et al., 1987; Peker et al., 2005; Roux et al., 1996; Solero et al., 1989). In Grade I meningiomas, there was no correlation between the histological subtype and patient outcome (Gezen et al., 2000; Gottfried et al., 2003; King et al., 1998; Klekamp et al., 1993; Levy et al., 1982; Namer et al., 1987; Peker et al., 2005; Roux et al., 1996; Solero et al., 1989). In this study, the most frequent histological type was clear cell meningioma. Clear cell meningioma of the spinal canal shows a tendency to occur in the lower thoracic, lumbar, or lumbosacral regions. A family history has been reported (Heth et al., 2000; Maxwell et al., 1998). Often they are noted at surgery to have no dural attachment (Holtzman et al., 1996; Maxwell et al., 1998; Mizutani et al., 2002; Zorludemir et al., 1995). They also have a peculiar age distribution with a significant number identified in childhood (Carra et al., 2001; Dubois et al., 1998; Heth et al., 2000; Zorludemir et al., 1995). Clear cell meningiomas are sparsely reported aggressive variants with a predilection for the cauda equina. In contrast to encapsulated meningiomas, clear cell variants often afflict a younger patient population, markedly recur after gross total resection, and metastasize. They are immunohistochemically distinct and can be discriminated from other primary and clear cell tumors through positive vimentin and epithelial membrane antigen staining (Liu et al., 2005).

7. Surgical treatment

7.1 Surgical approach

Treatment of lumbar spinal meningioma is predominantly surgical. The approach should allow sufficiently wide exposure of the tumor and the dural attachment. The most frequent approach has been posterior, by laminectomy at one level or by hemilaminectomy at one or two levels with lateral extension when necessary. In our series, a posterior approach was used in all but one case in which a combined approach (posterior-anterior-posterior) was used (Lee et al., 2002). In the majority of patients, it is possible to resect even large tumors safely and without causing spinal instability using a standard posterior or posterior-lateral laminectomy approach.

7.2 Tumor resection

The primary goal of surgery is complete safe tumor removal and decompression of the spinal cord or cauda equina. The dural attachment was coagulated in most cases in the reported studies (15% - 89%), and resection of the dural attachment was performed with suturing of a patch graft in 14% - 57% of cases (Gezen et al., 2000; Gottfried et al., 2003; King et al., 1998; Klekamp et al., 1993; Levy et al., 1982; Namer et al., 1987; Peker et al., 2005; Roux et al., 1996; Solero et al., 1989). Some authors prefer to separate the outer and inner layers of the dura and resect the inner layer together with the tumor (Saito et al., 2001). In our series, there was one case report of lumbar metaplastic meningioma that was resected completely without dural reconstruction using this method (Hirabayashi et al., 2009).

7.3 Patient complications

In the reported series, morbidity and mortality rates for spinal meningiomas were low with mean values of 6.2% and 2.1%, respectively (Setzer et al., 2007). The most frequent complications included CSF leakage and wound infection, which occurred in 0% - 4% and 0% - 6% of cases, respectively (Gezen et al., 2000; Gottfried et al., 2003; King et al., 1998; Klekamp et al., 1993; Levy et al., 1982; Namer et al., 1987; Peker et al., 2005; Roux et al., 1996; Solero et al., 1989). Other less common complications were pulmonary embolism, pneumonia, and myocardial infarction. Increased surgical morbidity has been identified with resection of tumors of anterior location (Gezen et al., 2000; Roser et al., 2006; Roux et al., 1996), en plaque meningiomas (Caroli et al., 2004), clear cell meningiomas (Liu et al., 2005), and the presence of intratumoral calcifications (Roser et al., 2006; Roux et al., 1996).

Although there were 5 patients with clear cell meningioma and 1 patient with intratumoral calcification (Hirabayashi et al., 2009) in this series, there were no complications of surgery for lumbar spinal meningiomas.

7.4 Tumor recurrence

Tumor recurrence in Grade I spinal meningiomas is uncommon, with an incidence rate ranging from 0% to 14.7% in the reviewed studies (Gezen et al., 2000; Gottfried et al., 2003; King et al., 1998; Klekamp et al., 1993; Levy et al., 1982; Namer et al., 1987; Peker et al., 2005; Roux et al., 1996; Solero et al., 1989). Compared to other locations, the recurrence rate of spinal meningiomas is low (Mirimanoff et al., 1985). Very few patients with Grade II to IV spinal meningiomas were included in the reviewed studies, and thus a comparison between tumor grades and recurrence rates of spinal meningiomas was not possible. In one series, the total recurrence rate was 14.7%, which was presumably explained by the inclusion of a greater percentage of Grade II and III meningiomas (Cooper and Epstein., 1985). Tumor histology was metastatic meningioma from intracranial meningioma in 2 of 10 cases of tumor recurrence in this study.

7.5 Adjuvant therapies

Due to the good outcomes and low recurrence rates following surgical therapy, complete tumor resection is the best treatment for spinal meningiomas. In cases of subtotal resection, the efficacy of radiosurgery and stereotactic radiotherapy for intracranial meningiomas with low complication rates has been well established (Barami et al., 2007; Chang et al., 2001; Chin et al., 2003; Pollock, 2003). In this study, four of 9 patients were treated with radiotherapy. As subtotal resection will likely result in rapid tumor recurrence or progression (Prinz et al., 1996), radiotherapy may be considered in patients with subtotal lumbar spinal meningioma resection.

8. Conclusions

Due to the excellent outcome after surgery for benign lumbar spinal meningiomas together with the low complication rates, early diagnosis is required with surgery as the treatment of choice. The possibility of clear cell meningioma should be considered in young patients with lumbar or lumbosacral meningioma.

9. References

Albanese, V., & Platania, N. (2002). Spinal intradural extramedullary tumors. Personal experience. *J Neurosurg Sci.* Vol. 46, No. 1, (March 2002), pp. 18-24, ISSN 0390-5616

Barami, K., Grow, A., Brem, S., Dagnew, E., & Sloan, A.E. (2007). Vascular complications after radiosurgery for meningiomas. *Neurosurg Focus.* Vol. 22, No. 3, (2007), pp. E9, ISSN 1092-0684

Boet, R., Ng, H.K., Kumta, S., Chan, LC., Chiu, KW., & Poon, WS. (2004). Lumbosacral clear-cell meningioma treated with subtotal resection and radiotherapy. *J Clin Neurosci.* Vol. 11, No. 4, (May 2004), pp. 432-436, ISSN 0967-5868

Caroli, E., Acqui, M., Roperto, R., Ferrante, L., & D'Andrea, G. (2004). Spinal en plaque meningiomas: a contemporary experience. *Neurosurgery*. Vol. 55, No. 6, (December 2004), pp. 1275-1279; discussion 1279, ISSN 1524-4040

Carrà, S., Drigo, P., Gardiman, M., Perilongo, G., & Rigobello, L. (2001). Clear-cell meningioma in a 22-month-old male: a case report and literature review. *Pediatr Neurosurg*. Vol. 34, No. 5, (May 2001), pp. 264-267, ISSN 1016-2291

Chang, SD., & Adler, JR. (2001). Current status and optimal use of radiosurgery. *Oncology (Williston Park). Vol. 15, No. 2, (*February 2001), pp. 209-216; discussion 219-221, ISSN 0890-9091

Chen, M.H., Chen, S.J., & Lin, S.M. (2004). A lumbar clear cell meningioma with foraminal extension in a renal transplant recipient. *J Clin Neurosci*. Vol. 11, No. 6, (August 2004), pp. 665-667, ISSN 0967-5868

Chin, L.S., Szerlip, N.J., & Regine, W.F. (2003). Stereotactic radiosurgery for meningiomas. *Neurosurg Focus*. Vol. 14, No. 5, (May 2003), pp. e6, ISSN 1092-0684

Colen, C.B., Rayes, M., McClendon, J., Rabah, R., & Ham, S.D. (2009). Pediatric spinal clear cell meningioma. Case report. *J Neurosurg Pediatr*. Vol. 3, No. 1, (January 2009), pp. 57-60, ISSN 1933-0707

Conrad, M.D., Schonauer, C., Pelissou-Guyotat, I., Morel, C., Madarassy, G., & Deruty, R. (2001). Recurrent lumbosacral metastases from intracranial meningioma. Report of a case and review of the literature. *Acta Neurochir (Wien)*. Vol. 143, No. 9, (September 2001), pp. 935-937, ISSN 0001-6268

Cooper, P.R., & Epstein, F. (1985). Radical resection of intramedullary spinal cord tumors in adults. Recent experience in 29 patients. *J Neurosurg*. Vol. 63, No. 4, (October 1985), pp. 492-499, ISSN 0022-3085

Dubois, A., Sévely, A., Boetto, S., Delisle, M.B., & Manelfe, C. (1998). Clear-cell meningioma of the cauda equina. *Neuroradiology*. Vol. 40, No. 11, (November 1998), pp. 743-747, ISSN 0028-3940

Epstein, N.E., Drexler, S., & Schneider, J. (2005). Clear cell meningioma of the cauda equina in an adult: case report and literature review. *J Spinal Disord Tech*. Vol. 18, No. 6, (December 2005), pp. 539-543, ISSN 1536-0652

Gezen, F., Kahraman, S., Canakci, Z., & Bedük, A. (2000). Review of 36 cases of spinal cord meningioma. *Spine (Phila Pa 1976)*. Vol. 25, No. 6, (March 2000), pp. 727-731, ISSN 0362-2436

Gottfried, O.N., Gluf, W., Quinones-Hinojosa, A., Kan, P., & Schmidt, M.H. (2003). Spinal meningiomas: surgical management and outcome. *Neurosurg Focus*. Vol. 14, No. 6, (June 2003), pp. e2, ISSN 1092-0684

Helseth, A., & Mørk, S.J. (1989). Primary intraspinal neoplasms in Norway, 1955 to 1986. A population-based survey of 467 patients. *J Neurosurg*. Vol. 71, No. 6, (December 1989), pp. 842-845, ISSN 0022-3085

Heth, J.A., Kirby, P., & Menezes, A.H. (2000). Intraspinal familial clear cell meningioma in a mother and child. Case report. *J Neurosurg*, Vol. 93, No. 2 Suppl, (October 2000), pp. 317-321, ISSN 0022-3085

Hirabayashi, H., Takahashi, J., Kato, H., Ebara, S., & Takahashi, H. (2009). Surgical resection without dural reconstruction of a lumbar meningioma in an elderly woman. *Eur Spine J*. Vol. 18, No. Suppl 2 (July 2009), pp. 232-235, ISSN 1432-0932

Holtzman, R.N., & Jormark, S.C. (1996). Nondural-based lumbar clear cell meningioma. Case report. *J Neurosurg*. Vol. 84, No. 2, (February 1996), pp. 264-266, ISSN 0022-3085

King, A.T., Sharr, M.M., Gullan, R.W., & Bartlett, J.R. (1998). Spinal meningiomas: a 20-year review. *Br J Neurosurg*. Vol. 12, No. 6, (December 1998), pp. 521-526, ISSN 0268-8697

Klekamp, J., & Samii, M. (1999). Surgical results for spinal meningiomas. *Surg Neurol*. Vol. 52, No. 6, (December 1999), pp. 552-562, ISSN 0090-3019

Lee, Y.Y., Wen-Wei Hsu R., Huang, T.J., Hsueh, S., & Wang, J.Y. (2002). Metastatic meningioma in the sacrum: a case report. *Spine (Phila Pa 1976)*. Vol. 27, No. 4, (February 2002), pp. E100-103, ISSN 1528-1159

Levy, W.J., Bay, J., & Dohn, D. (1982). Spinal cord meningioma. *J Neurosurg*. Vol. 57, No. 6, (December 1982), pp. 804-812, ISSN 0022-3085

Liu, P.I., Liu, G.C., Tsai, K.B., Lin, C.L., & Hsu, J.S. (2005). Intraspinal clear-cell meningioma: case report and review of literature. *Surg Neurol*. Vol. 63, No. 3, (March 2005), pp. 285-288; discussion 288-289, ISSN 0090-3019

Maxwell, M., Shih, S.D., Galanopoulos, T., Hedley-Whyte, E.T., & Cosgrove, G.R. (1998). Familial meningioma: analysis of expression of neurofibromatosis 2 protein Merlin. Report of two cases. *J Neurosurg*. Vol. 88, No. 3, (March 1998), pp. 562-569, ISSN 0022-3085

McCormick, P.C., Post, K.D., & Stein, B.M. (1990). Intradural extramedullary tumors in adults. *Neurosurg Clin N Am*. Vol. 1, No. 3, (July 1990), pp. 591-608, ISSN 1042-3680

Mirimanoff, R.O., Dosoretz, D.E., Linggood, R.M., Ojemann, R.G., & Martuza, R.L. (1985). Meningioma: analysis of recurrence and progression following neurosurgical resection. *J Neurosurg*. Vol. 62, No. 1, (January 1985), pp. 18-24, ISSN 0022-3085

Mizutani, J., Fukuoka, M., Tsubouchi, S., Otsuka, T., Tono, Y., Shimizu, S., & Matsui, N. (2002). A rare case of lumbosacral meningioma: nondural attachment and possible enlargement by orally administered sex steroid. *Spine (Phila Pa 1976)*. Vol. 27, No. 16, (August 2002), pp. E377-381, ISSN 1528-1159

Namer, I.J., Pamir, M.N., Benli, K., Saglam, S., & Erbengi, A. (1987). Spinal meningiomas. *Neurochirurgia (Stuttg)*. Vol. 30, No. 1, (January 1987), pp. 11-15, ISSN 0028-3819

Oviedo, A., Pang, D., Zovickian, J., & Smith, M. (2005). Clear cell meningioma: case report and review of the literature. *Pediatr Dev Pathol*. Vol. 8, No. 3, (May-June 2005), pp. 386-390, ISSN 1093-5266

Parsa, A.T., Lee, J., Parney, I.F., Weinstein, P., McCormick, P.C., & Ames, C. (2004). Spinal cord and intradural-extraparenchymal spinal tumors: current best care practices and strategies. *J Neurooncol*. Vol. 69, No. 1-3, (August-September 2004), pp. 291-318, ISSN 0167-594X

Peker, S., Cerçi, A., Ozgen, S., Isik, N., Kalelioglu, M., & Pamir, M.N. (2005) Spinal meningiomas: evaluation of 41 patients. *J Neurosurg Sci*. Vol. 49, No. 1, (March 2005), pp. 7-11, ISSN 0390-5616

Pollock, B.E. (2003). Stereotactic radiosurgery for intracranial meningiomas: indications and results. *Neurosurg Focus*. Vol. 14, No. 5, (May 2003), pp. e4, ISSN 1092-0684

Prinz, M., Patt, S., Mitrovics, T., & Cervós-Navarro, J. (1996). Clear cell meningioma: report of a spinal case. *Gen Diagn Pathol*. Vol. 141, No. 3-4, (March 1996), pp. 261-267, ISSN 0947-823X

Roser, F., Nakamura, M., Bellinzona, M., Ritz, R., Ostertag, H., & Tatagiba, M.S. (2006). Proliferation potential of spinal meningiomas. *Eur Spine J.* Vol. 15, No. 2, (February 2006), pp. 211-215, ISSN 0940-6719

Roux, F.X., Nataf, F., Pinaudeau, M., Borne, G., Devaux, B., & Meder, J.F. (1996). Intraspinal meningiomas: review of 54 cases with discussion of poor prognosis factors and modern therapeutic management. *Surg Neurol.* Vol. 46, No. 5, (Nov 1996), pp. 458-463; discussion 463-454, ISSN 0090-3019

Saito, T., Arizono, T., Maeda, T., Terada, K., & Iwamoto, Y. (2001). A novel technique for surgical resection of spinal meningioma. *Spine (Phila Pa 1976).* Vol. 26, No. 16, (Aug 2001), pp. 1805-1808, ISSN 0362-2436

Schroth, G., Thron, A., Guhl, L., Voigt, K., Niendorf, H.P., & Garces, L.R. (1987). Magnetic resonance imaging of spinal meningiomas and neurinomas. Improvement of imaging by paramagnetic contrast enhancement. *J Neurosurg.* Vol. 66, No. 5, (May 1987), pp. 695-700, ISSN 0022-3085

Setzer, M., Vatter, H., Marquardt, G., Seifert, V., & Vrionis, F.D. (2007). Management of spinal meningiomas: surgical results and a review of the literature. *Neurosurg Focus.* Vol. 23, No. 4, (2007), pp. E14, ISSN 1092-0684

Solero, C.L., Fornari, M., Giombini, S., Lasio, G., Oliveri, G., Cimino, C., & Pluchino, F. (1989). Spinal meningiomas: review of 174 operated cases. *Neurosurgery.* Vol. 25, No. 2, (August 1989), pp. 153-160, ISSN 0148-396X

Traul, D.E., Shaffrey, M.E., & Schiff, D. (2007) Part I: spinal-cord neoplasms-intradural neoplasms. *Lancet Oncol.* Vol. 8, No. 1, (January 2007), pp. 35-45, ISSN 1470-2045

Tredway, T.L., Santiago, P., Hrubes, M.R., Song, J.K., Christie, S.D., & Fessler, R.G. (2006). Minimally invasive resection of intradural-extramedullary spinal neoplasms. *Neurosurgery.* Vol. 58, No. 1 Suppl 1, (February 2006), pp. ONS52-58; discussion ONS52-58, ISSN 1524-4040

Van Goethem, J.W., van den Hauwe, L., Ozsarlak, O., De Schepper, A.M., & Parizel, P.M. (2004). Spinal tumors. *Eur J Radiol.* Vol. 50, No. 2, (May 2004), pp. 159-176, ISSN 0720-048X

Voulgaris, S., Alexiou, G.A., Mihos, E., Karagiorgiadis, D., Zigouris, A., Fotakopoulos, G., Drosos, D., & Pahaturidis, D. (2010). Posterior approach to ventrally located spinal meningiomas. *Eur Spine J.* Vol. 19, No. 7, (July 2010), pp. 1195-1199, ISSN 1432-0932

Zorludemir, S., Scheithauer, B.W., Hirose, T., Van Houten, C., Miller, G., & Meyer, F.B. (1995). Clear cell meningioma. A clinicopathologic study of a potentially aggressive variant of meningioma. *Am J Surg Pathol.* Vol. 19, No. 5, (May 1995), pp. 493-505, ISSN 0147-5185

3

Radiation Therapy in the Management of Meningiomas

Frederik Vernimmen
University College Cork
Ireland

1. Introduction

Although most meningiomas are benign, they have a surprisingly wide spectrum of clinical and histological characteristics. The WHO classification attempts to better predict the spectrum of clinical characteristics with a histological grading system based on statistically significant clinical-pathological correlations (1). There are three types of meningiomas in this classification; benign (WHO grade I), atypical (WHO grade II) and anaplastic (malignant; WHO grade III). Because the majority of meningiomas, 80%, fall under grade I (1), they are the ones on which the most literature is available. For grade I lesions, complete surgical removal results in a permanent cure in a high percentage of patients. However the anatomic localization of meningiomas, such as at the skull base, can make complete surgery difficult, and gross total resection only, results in control rates that vary from 44% to 90% and carry a high risk of neurologic morbidity . When surgery is incomplete, the recurrence rate is high, and patients suffer long-term morbidity, decreased survival, and the risk of histological dedifferentiation (2-7).

Radiation is well established as a treatment modality to control meningiomas, and can be used for: a) irresectable lesions, b) in patients to whom the risks of a resection are unacceptable, c) inoperable patients, and d) for recurrence or incomplete resection (8-13).

1.1 Diagnosis

The diagnosis usually comes after investigations for neurological complaints, but is also regularly made during imaging of the brain for other reasons. The diagnosis is finalized by the obtaining of histology. Offering the patient surgery for the sole purpose of obtaining histology can sometimes be debatable. This is particularly the case in skull base meningiomas, where the chances of complete removal without additional morbidity are slim and when no debulking is required. In such a scenario it is acceptable to go by the classic clinical picture and the typical radiological characteristics of benign meningiomas, to make the diagnosis (14). However good clinical judgement is required in order to suspect the possibility of a more sinister type of lesion.

2. Radiation therapy

Irradiation is the deposition of energy (dose) in the target by various radiation modalities using a variety of irradiation techniques. This dose is expressed in units of Gray (Gy), and the beam energy used to deliver the dose is expressed as Mega Volts (MV). It is the absorption of this energy by the cell structures that causes the individual cell damage resulting in control of the disease. The cell damage is on the DNA of the cells. This damage is either direct or indirect, ionizing the atoms which make up the DNA chain. Indirect ionization happens as a result of the ionization of water molecules, forming free radicals, notably hydroxyl radicals. These are "chemically aggressive" compounds which when formed in close proximity to the DNA molecules damage the DNA. Most of the radiation effect is through these free radicals. They cause single and double strand breaks in the DNA. Cells have mechanisms for repairing DNA damage, but double-stranded DNA breaks are difficult to repair and are the most significant way by which cell death occurs. Cancer cells generally are undifferentiated and stem cell-like, they reproduce more, and have a diminished ability to repair sub-lethal damage compared to most healthy differentiated cells. This DNA damage is then passed on through cell division, accumulating damage to the cancer cell's DNA, and causing them to die or reproduce more slowly.

One of the major limitations of photon radiation therapy is that the cells of solid tumors become deficient in oxygen. Solid tumors can outgrow their blood supply, causing a low-oxygen state known as hypoxia. Oxygen is a potent radio sensitizer, increasing the effectiveness of a given dose of radiation by forming DNA damaging free radicals. Tumor cells in a hypoxic environment may be as much as 2 to 3 times more resistant to radiation damage than those in a normal oxygen environment. In the case of meningiomas, seeing that they are usually very vascular lesions this oxygen effect is not a major factor in their treatment with ionizing radiation.

Direct damage to cancer cell DNA occurs through high-LET (linear energy transfer) charged particles irradiation such as with proton, carbon or neon ions which have an antitumor effect which is independent of tumor oxygen supply because these particles act mostly via direct energy transfer usually causing double-stranded DNA breaks. Due to their relatively large mass, protons and other charged particles have little lateral side scatter in the tissue; the beam does not broaden much, hence stays focused on the tumor shape and delivers small dose side-effects to surrounding tissue. These particles can be charged to different levels of energy providing the required tissue penetration to reach the tumor. This reduces damage to healthy tissue between the charged particle radiation source and the tumor and sets a finite range for tissue damage after the tumor has been reached. No energy is deposited beyond the point of the calculated depth penetration saving normal tissue from the radiation effects.

2.1 Dose calculations

Before treatment, a CT scan is performed with the patients head immobilized by either a cast made from a thermoplastic material or by a stereotactic frame directly fixated to the patient's skull. The ability to import other images such as MRI scans into the planning system, a technique called image fusion , allows to identify the tumor and surrounding normal structures with great accuracy.

The delivery parameters of a prescribed dose are determined during treatment planning (part of dosimetry). Treatment planning is generally performed on dedicated computers using specialized treatment planning software. Depending on the radiation delivery method, several beam angles may be used to sum the total necessary dose. The planner will try to design a plan that delivers a uniform prescription dose to the tumor and minimizes dose to surrounding healthy tissues.

2.2 Radiation equipment

2.2.1 Photon (gamma ray) therapy

A number of radiation therapy machines are available; the most commonly used are the one's using gamma rays (photons) to deliver the therapeutic dose. The Gamma Knife®, Cyberknife®, and the linear accelerator (Linac) fall in this category. In addition a small linear accelerator used in a rotational way around the patient (Tomotherapy) is also available.

With the *gamma knife*, multiple small static beams, each produced by individual Cobalt sources are directed to a fixed single spot or isocenter. This area of convergence of all the small beams can be placed in multiple locations within the target volume by moving the patient's head around with small movements of the head fixation mechanism.

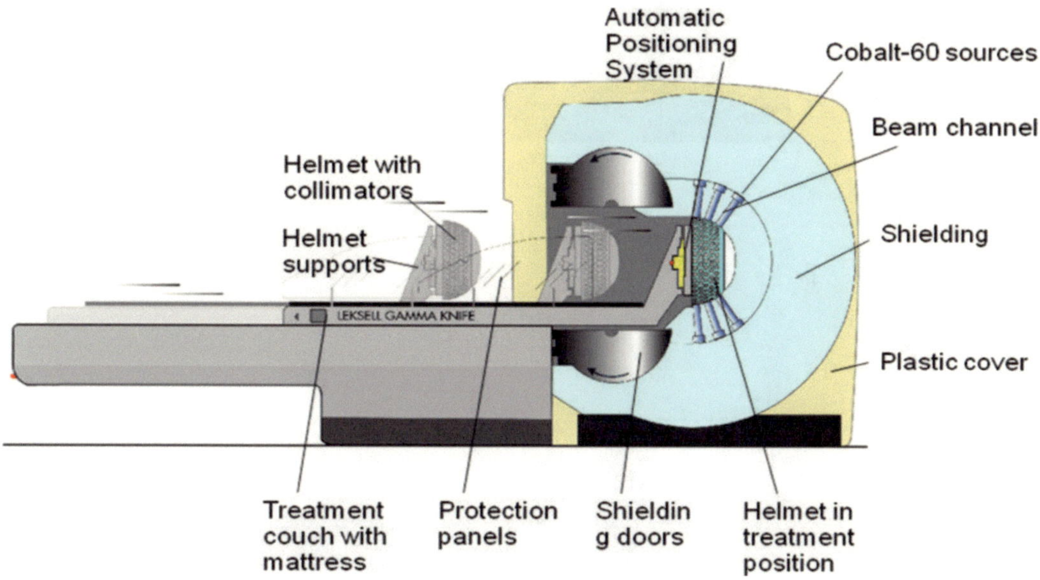

Fig. 1.

With the *linear accelerator* (Fig 2a) the beams are directed at an isocenter, which is in a fixed position in the treatment room and which can be placed in the target volume and shifted around if necessary by moving the couch onto which the patient is lying. Rotation of the gantry, which produces the beam, around this isocenter, together with a couch rotation, provides for a number of individually shaped beams coming from different directions allowing full coverage of the target volume. For stereotactic irradiation additional beam collimation is provided by either a set of cones or by a micro multileaf collimator (Fig 2b). These devices are not part of the standard equipment and have to be acquired separately.

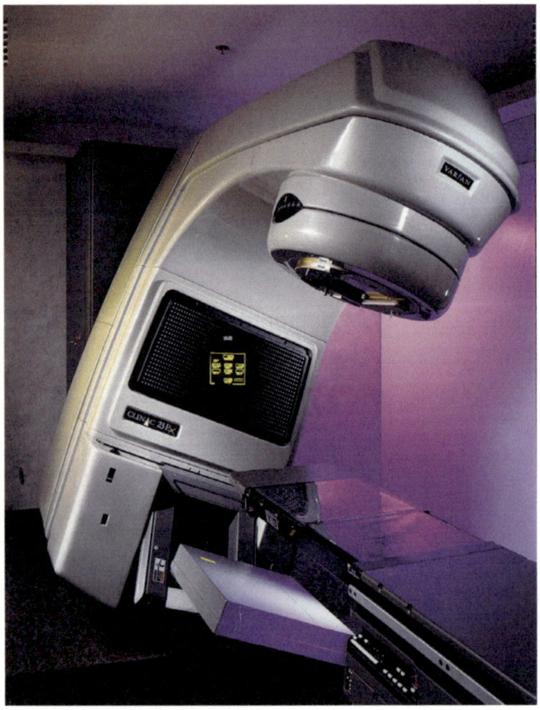

Fig. 2a.

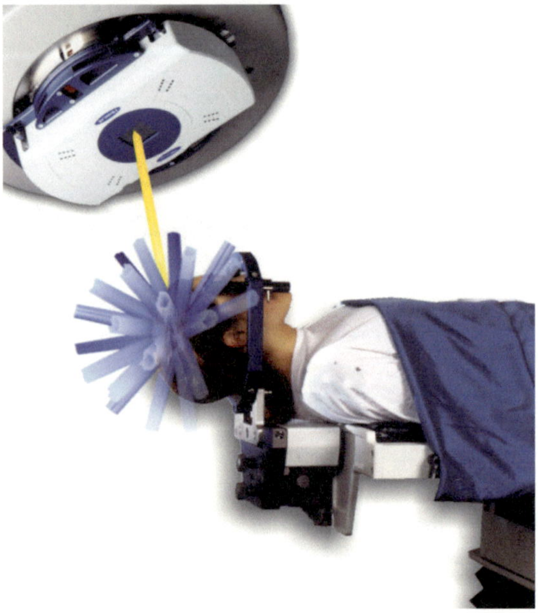

Fig. 2b.

A large body of literature exists for both these techniques in the management of meningiomas

The *Cyberknife®* uses a small linear accelerator supported by a robot arm. This in conjunction with the use of a robotic couch supporting the patient allows for numerous small beams to come in from a large variety of angles. The "cross firing "of these multiple small beams through the target results in the full dose been given to the whole target volume.

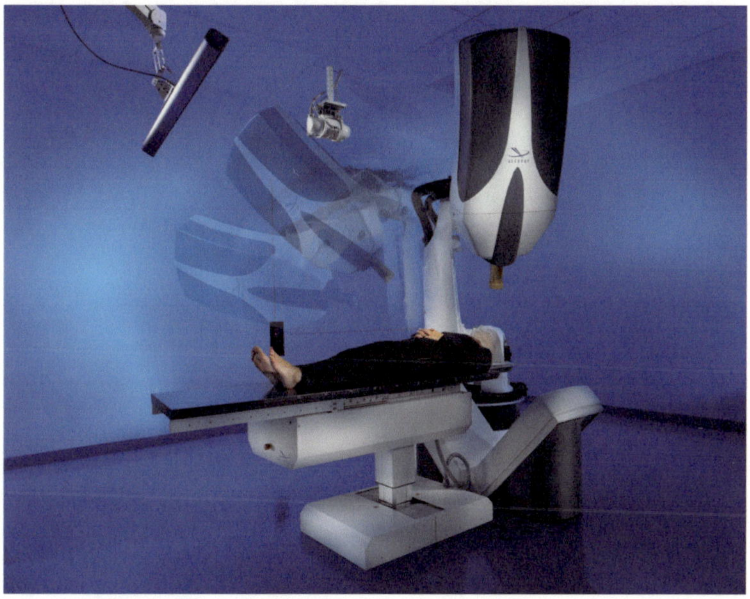

Fig. 3.

Tomotherapy® is very similar in its concept to the use of helical CT-scanning in diagnostic imaging. A narrow beam is rotating through the target whilst the couch onto which the patient is lying is moving perpendicular to the plane of rotation. This technique is mainly used to deliver intensity modulated radiotherapy (IMRT) and limited literature is available concerning its use for intracranial meningiomas (15).

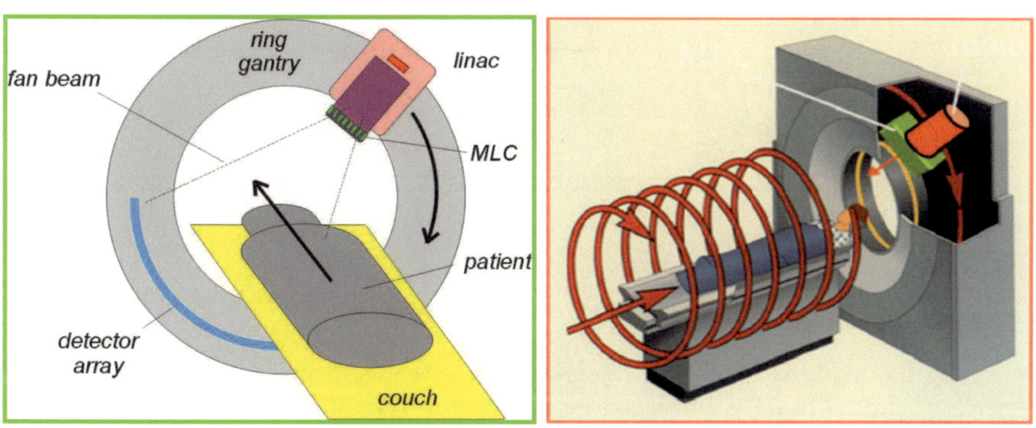

Fig. 4.

All the above techniques use photons, also called gamma rays, to deliver the dose.

The radiation equipment is housed in a treatment unit bunker, whose purpose is to protect the staff and members of the public from the radiation. A typical bunker for a linear accelerator is illustrated. Requirements for a bunker include walls and a roof both of a thickness offering sufficient protection, high density concrete without joints or air pockets and a 'maze' design to reduce the radiation dose reaching the door of the bunker or vault.

2.2.2 Bunker

The wall and roof thickness is determined by the energy (the penetration power) of the radiation. For cobalt sourced radiation the concrete thickness should be approximately 80 cm. For linear accelerators the thickness varies between 2 and 3 meters for covering the range of low, medium and high-energy linear accelerators.

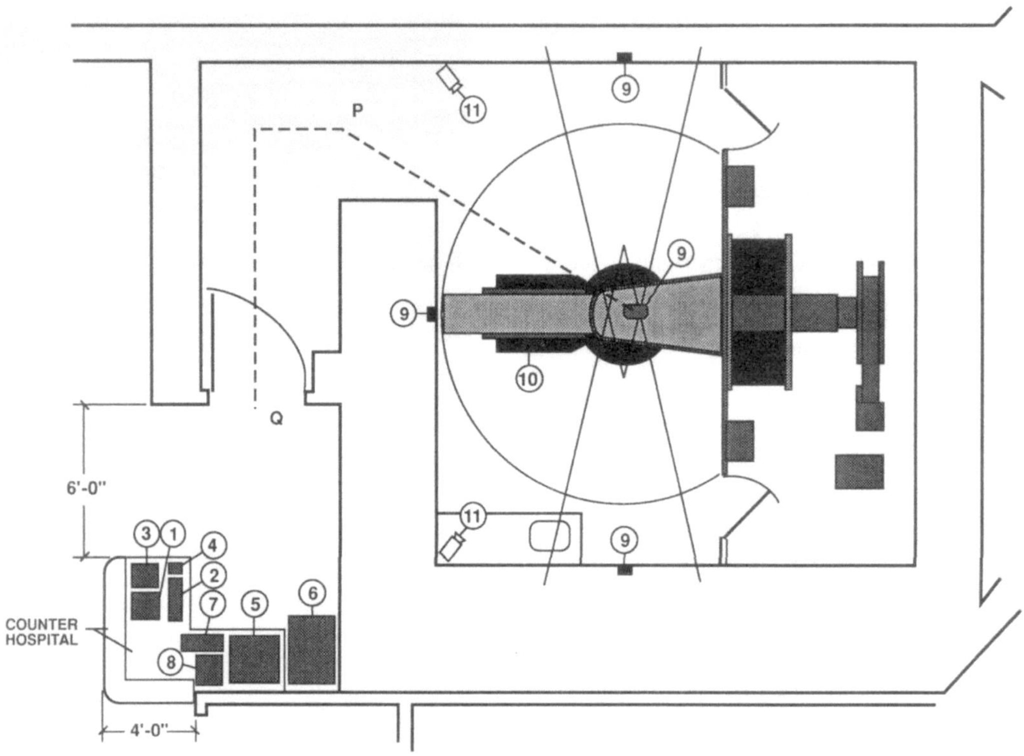

2.2.3 Charged particle therapy

Delivering the required dose with charged particle beams, mainly proton beams, is also possible. A proton beam is produced by a cyclotron (Fig 5b) or a synchrotron and has particular physical characteristics (the Bragg peak) which make it theoretically a better radiation modality in and around sensitive structures such as the brain as there is no dose distal to the peak and a lower dose proximal to the target (Fig 5a).

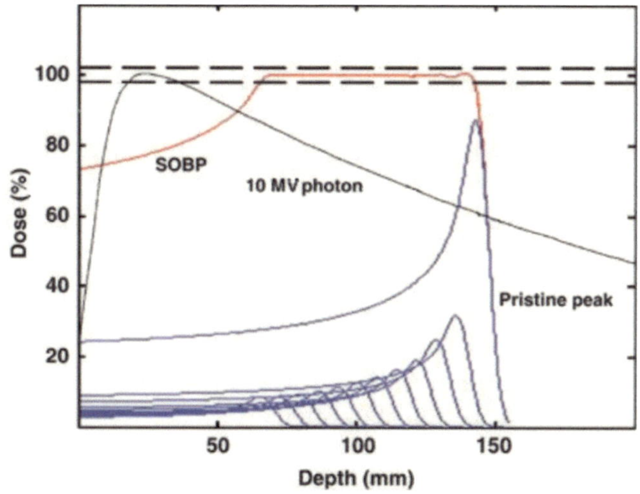

Fig. 5a.

The primary narrow beam leaving the cyclotron or synchrotron is scattered to provide a beam of sufficient size for clinical use. Because the peak is usually to narrow to cover the length of the target volume along the beam axis, this peak needs to be spread out over the full distance of the target in order to cover it with the full dose. This dose delivery technique is referred to as a Spread Out Bragg Peak (SOBP) (16,17). In more and more centres, the primary proton beam is not scattered, but used in a spot scanning mode, whereby the target volume is covered by multiple scanned "spots". This technique allows for a better dose distribution, but is more complex to deliver and to verify. The availability of proton therapy facilities worldwide is however still limited. The availability of other charged particle beams, such as Carbon ions and Helium ions is even more limited. They have the additional advantage over protons in that they cause more radiobiological damage per unit of dose. In other words their Radiobiological Effect (RBE) is higher (18).

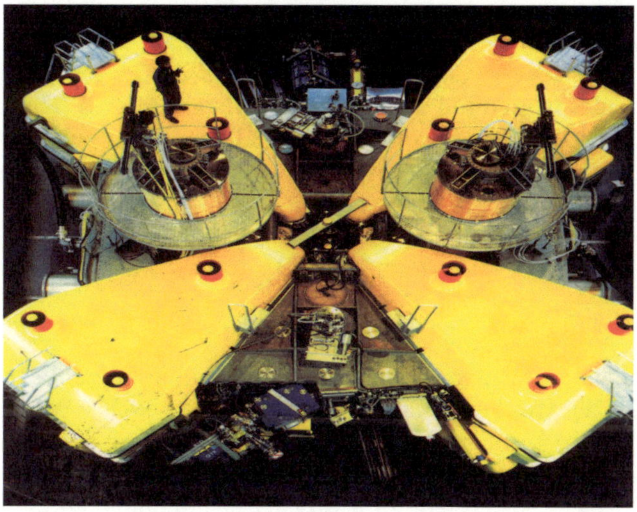

Fig. 5b.

2.3 Irradiation techniques

Technically the radiation can be administered in a variety of ways:

a. *Conventional* 3 dimensional (3-D) way. The patient's head is immobilized by a cast and images are acquired for planning. A number of beams coming from various angles are directed at the target, but the overall geometric accuracy of the treatment set up is less then for a stereotactic technique, and the dose gradient is also less steep. The 3-D technique is however available in most radiotherapy departments.
b. *Intensity-modulated radiation therapy* (IMRT) is an advanced type of high-precision radiation that is the next generation of 3DCRT. IMRT also improves the ability to conform the treatment volume to concave tumor shapes, for example when the tumor is wrapped around a vulnerable structure such as the spinal cord or a major organ or blood vessel. The pattern of radiation delivery is determined using highly tailored computing applications to perform optimization and treatment simulation. The radiation dose is consistent with the 3-D shape of the tumor by controlling, or modulating, the radiation beam's intensity. The radiation dose intensity is elevated near the gross tumor volume while radiation among the neighboring normal tissue is decreased or avoided completely. The customized radiation dose is intended to maximize tumor dose while simultaneously protecting the surrounding normal tissue. This may result in better tumor targeting, lessened side effects, and improved treatment outcomes than even 3DCRT. This technique is finding its way into stereotactic radiation
c. *Stereotactically*; this is a technique for precisely directing the beams of radiation in three planes using x-y-z coordinates in order to target a specific locus in the head, with a geometric accuracy of ≤1 mm. This requires accurate immobilisation of the head with either a stereotactic frame fixed to the patient's skull or a well constructed cast, made of some form of thermo plastic material, completely encasing patient's head. With the immobilization device in place, MRI and CT-scan images are acquired for delineating the target and surrounding structures, and for the dose calculations, using specialized dose calculation soft ware. The precise dose delivery along with the presence of very steep dose gradients in all three dimensions facilitates the treatment of target volumes to a high dose while maintaining the dose to the adjacent healthy tissue within the accepted tolerance levels. Careful verification of the target position by advanced imaging techniques is required prior to each radiation session. This technique requires additional infrastructure on top of the normal Linac equipment and is not always available in every radiotherapy department.

The technological progress in equipment is leading to an ever increasing overlap of these techniques.

2.4 Radiobiology

The linear quadratic model is the mathematical model that best describes the biological effect of radiation on cells (19). This biological effect can be expressed as a Biological Effective Dose (BED), and is given by the formula: BED= total dose (1+ dose per fraction/ alpha-beta).Various radiation schedules can be compared with each other by calculating their respective Bed's. For this, the α/β value which is a constant for a very specific radiation effect on a specific type of tissue, needs to be known (20). Knowing the α/ß value for a specific effect on a specific target tissue is useful for the following reasons: 1) It allows for more accurate calculations of biological equivalent fractionation schedules; 2) The α/ß value gives an indication of what sort of a fractionation schedule would be beneficial in terms of therapeutic gain; 3) It allows one to determine the minimum number of fractions required in order to keep a critical structure within tolerance when this critical structure is in close proximity to the target

For histological benign radiosurgical targets information on α/ß ratios is very limited , but in general low α/ß ratios have been assumed, based on the clinical and radiological observation that these targets are slow growing.

For radiological control of histological benign meningiomas (Grade I) this value has been estimated at 3.7 Gy (21). Normal tissue has an α/β in the range of 2-3 Gy (19). This small difference between the α/ß values of normal surrounding tissue versus the target tissue theoretically allows for an increase in the differential radiation effect on both these tissues by increasing the number of fractions, this is called therapeutic gain (21,22,23,27). Most of this gain is achieved by going from 1 fraction to about 7-9 fractions and than flattens off going to 25-30 fractions.

3. Total dose/fractionation schedules

For a standard radiation course, the total dose is fractionated (spread out over time) for several important reasons. Fractionation allows normal cells time to recover, while tumor cells are generally less efficient in repair between fractions. Fractionation also allows tumor cells that were in a relatively radio-resistant phase of the cell cycle during one treatment to cycle into a sensitive phase of the cycle before the next fraction is given. Similarly, tumor cells that were chronically or acutely hypoxic (and therefore more radioresistant) may reoxygenate between fractions, improving the tumor cell kill. A typical fractionation schedule for adults is 1.8 to 2 Gy per day, five days a week, for 6 - 7 weeks, i.e. doses in the order of 60 - 70 Gy. For meningiomas, the radiation dose/fractionation schedules used vary. When the total dose is delivered in 1 single session (fraction), this is defined as stereotactic radiosurgery (SRS). Using a small number of fractions (3-7) is called hypofractionated radiotherapy which is commonly applied under stereotactic conditions and hence is called Hypo Fractionated Stereotactic Radiotherapy (HSRT). A conventional fractionation schedule of 25-30 fractions can be used based on 3-D conformal techniques, but is called Fractionated Stereotactic Radiotherapy (FSRT) if all the fractions are delivered under stereotactic conditions. The majority of lesions have historically been treated with SRS, or 3-D RT, and the literature on results with HSRT is still limited.

4. Intracranial meningiomas

1. Grade I meningiomas

Radiation therapy can be used very successfully as the sole modality for unresectable or inoperable lesions. After partial removal serious consideration should be given to offer the patient post operative radiotherapy and radiation should definitely be considered in the management of post surgical recurrences.

There are no major differences in overall results when comparing SRS ⇔ HSRT ⇔ FSRT (table I). For SRS, minimum target doses, covering the surface of the lesion, fall in the range of 13 - 16 Gy (10,11,12,13,14,16, 24).

Author	Total dose/Gy	Fractionation	Radiological control	Complications
Flickinger, et al. (14)	14	SRS	93% -10 years	8.8%
Lo, et al. (33)	14	SRS	93% - 3 years	6%
	54	FSRT	93.3% - 3 years	5.5%
Roche, et al. (53)	13	SRS	100% - 4 years	6%
Pollock, et al. (54)	16	SRS	94% - 3 years	8%
Selch, et al. (55)	50.4	FSRT	97% - 3 years	0%
Villavincencio, et al. (56)	15	SRS	95% - 5 years	9%
Vernimmen, et al. (57)	24.8 *	HSRT	88% - 3 years	5.5%
Debus, et al. (58)	56.8	FSRT	97% - 5 years	1.6%
Mahadevan, et al. (59)	25 – 30	HSRT	100% - 2 years	0%
Torres, et al. (60)	15.7	SRS	90% - 3.5 years	5%
	48.4	FSRT	97.2% - 2 years	5.2%
Spiegelmann, et al. (61)	13.5	SRS	98% - 5.5years	4.9%
Zada, et al. (62)	16	SRS	94% - 6 years	8%

* proton beam therapy

Table 1.

For HSRT, total doses in the region of 24 - 40 Gy, given in 3- 5 fractions have been used (18,51). FSRT doses fall in the range of 50 -56 Gy at 1.8 to 2 Gy per fraction.

The question therefore is what is the most appropriate dose/fractionation schedule? Factors that influence the decision are:

a. Volume and shape of the lesion:

Although no absolute guidelines exist in general one can state that as the volume of the lesion increases it becomes more and more difficult to safely offer the patient SRS (25,26,28). As a general rule lesions with a diameter ≤ then 2.5 – 3.0 cm are suitable for SRS. A complex shape of the lesion, which can happen with lesions of the skull base, can also, apart from volume restrictions, give sometimes limitations for the use of SRS (28). Here the different irradiation techniques have slight advantages and disadvantages (29).

Larger volume or complex shaped lesions can be treated with FSRT or HSRT. HSRT has the advantage of an overall shorter treatment time.

b. Proximity of critical normal structures:

Peripheral nerves have a fairly good resistance to radiation induced damage (30); hence the cranial nerves III - XII are usually not a major dose limiting factor. However the optic apparatus and especially the optic chiasma are vulnerable to radiation induced damage due to the late side effects of radiation therapy (31). So even for small lesions in very close proximity to the optic chiasma, FSRT or HSRT might be indicated as fractionation helps in improving the tolerance of the chiasma and other normal surrounding structures. The brain or brainstem are normally not directly invaded by Grade I and II meningiomas, hence there is no need to include them in the target volume. However when close contact exists they can receive a significant dose. Therefore "debulking" surgery with the aim of not only reducing the overall volume, but more importantly to increase the space between the meningioma and the normal tissues can be very valuable. In view of the very rapid dose fall off outside the target volume possible with stereotactic techniques, even a small gain in distance can reduce the dose to the normal structure considerable and hence reduce the chance of late damaging effects.

When a critical structure is totally or partially encased by the meningioma a strong point can be made for FSRT on *radiobiological grounds*. Full fractionation offers the best compromise between disease control and late normal tissue damage.

In a situation of close proximity, and when SRS is deemed not feasible, a hypofractionated schedule (HSRT) should be considered. When there is still concern for late reactions with HSRT or when the disease encases a sensitive structure fully fractionated therapy is required (32,33).

2. Grade II meningiomas

The best treatment protocol for this group is still not clear. In terms of dose/fractionation schedule most centres use the same as for grade I meningiomas. The same dose/fractionation selection factors as for grade I meningiomas apply. It is only their increased propensity to recur that would indicate a more aggressive use of radiation therapy in the post operative situation (34,35,36,37).

3. Grade III meningiomas

Considered malignant in terms of their histology and clinical behaviour they have a high mitotic index. Hence they should be treated as malignancies, with post operative radiation indicated even for completely excised lesions (38). As they can invade surrounding structures, inclusion of some surrounding normal tissue in the target volume is often necessary. This, plus the fact that they are likely to have a high α/ß ratio in the order of 10 Gy (23) requires the use of fully fractionated therapy in the order of 56 - 60 Gy in 28- 30 fractions to obtain the best possible results.

5. Results

5.1 Disease control

In evaluating the results of different treatment modalities for meningiomas, it is important to clearly define the end point. For histological benign lesions one expects the lesion to have disappeared radiologically after complete surgical resection. On the other hand, after primary radiation therapy the lesion rarely disappears completely. However, if after radiation therapy, a lesion remains radiologically stable for many years, and there is no progression of the clinical picture, the patient can be considered cured. Radiological follow up post radiotherapy usually reveals a small to moderate shrinkage of the lesion and a decrease in contrast enhancement. Often patients obtain some improvement of clinical neurological symptoms (39). This clinical improvement can happen without obvious radiological improvement. When used as a primary modality alone, several studies have shown a radiological control in the order of 88 - 100% and a clinical improvement or stable clinical picture in the order of 87-100% (Table I).

Fewer studies are available for the less benign histology's. This is because meningiomas need long term follow up to assess their response to therapy and most study's with long term follow up were based on the old classification. Of note is that whereas in the old classification about 5% of cases were classified as atypical meningiomas, in the current 2007 WHO classification, about 20-35% are classified grade II (40). Atypical meningiomas have a higher propensity to recur (1). Although the role of post operative radiotherapy for completely removed lesions is not well defined, in cases were there is residual disease post operatively, radiotherapy is advisable (41,42,43).

5.2 Side effects

Radiation therapy is in itself painless. Radiation side effects are classified as acute (during treatment) or late, with the late effects presenting themselves many months or years after the radiation was delivered. The nature, severity, and longevity of side effects depends on the organs that receive the radiation, the treatment itself (type of radiation, dose, fractionation), and the patient. Most side effects are predictable and expected. Side effects from radiation are usually limited to the area of the patient's body that is under treatment. One of the aims of modern radiation therapy is to reduce side effects to a minimum, and to help the patient to understand and to deal with those side effects which are unavoidable.

5.2.1 Acute effects

Side effects during therapy are minimal and are usually related to the patients head immobilisation system, and area of brain involved. Even a low dose on the brainstem can cause nausea, and localized headache can occur at the site of the meningeal involvement. The normal brain, connective tissues and the meningioma are late responding tissues (low $\alpha/ß$ values) and hence very little acute effects tend to occur during the course of the radiotherapy. Other side effects are fatigue and skin irritation, like a mild to moderate sun burn. During a fully fractionated radiation course, the fatigue often sets in during the middle of the course and can last for weeks after treatment ends. The irradiated skin will heal, but may not be as elastic as it was before. However as the field sizes used in stereotactic irradiation are usually very small compared to conventional radiation for malignancies the areas of skin affected are minimal.

5.2.2 Late side effects

More important are the late side effects which when they occur can either be transient and improve or become permanent. Late side effects occur months to years after treatment and are generally limited to the area that has been treated. They are often due to damage of blood vessels and connective tissue cells. The seriousness of many late effects are reduced by fractionation.

Most commonly oedema of the surrounding brain is noted on radiological imaging which might or might not be symptomatic (44). Para falx meningiomas have a higher propensity to develop surrounding brain oedema. This might be related to the fact that they tend to have a large contact zone with the surrounding brain in comparison with skull base meningiomas (44,45). The incidence of late effects on cranial nerves is low. Overall the incidence of side effects varies around 3- 6% (28,30,46,47).

Fibrosis: Tissues which have been irradiated tend to become less elastic over time due to a diffuse scarring process.

Epilation may occur on any hair bearing skin. It only occurs within the radiation field. Hair loss may be permanent with a single dose of 10 Gy, but if the dose is fractionated permanent hair loss may not occur until dose exceeds 45 Gy.

Cognitive decline is definitely a side effect that occurs when the whole brain or large parts of the brain are irradiated, such as in the case of whole brain irradiation for multiple brain metastasis or large brain tumors. For large meningiomas this is a factor to take into consideration in the decision on the use of radiation therapy. For small volume stereotactic irradiation the effect on cognition is not well established, but presumed to be minimal, and will primarily depend on the area of brain involved. In middle aged or elderly people it is difficult to distinguish between normal aging processes versus a radiation induced effect. Prospective studies are required to address this issue.

Carcinogenesis; Radiation is a potential cause of cancer, and secondary malignancies are seen in a very small minority of patients - usually less than 1/1000. It usually occurs 20 - 30 years following treatment. In the vast majority of cases, this risk is greatly outweighed by the benefit of the proposed radiation therapy. In elderly patients carcinogenesis is of less a concern in view of the long latent time. However the use of radiation for benign lesions like meningiomas in young people causes more concern and should definitely be addressed in the discussion on treatment options with the patient.

6. Spinal canal meningiomas

Adult primary spinal cord tumours represent 2% to 4% of all central nervous system neoplasms and of these meningiomas constitute about 25% (48, 49). Hence very few centres can report on the results exclusively for spinal meningiomas. Surgery is the main stay for managing these lesions as the spinal cord and the meningioma have an intricate anatomical relation, with spinal cord compression always a possibility if not already present at time of presentation. Spinal meningiomas are separated from the spinal cord by a discrete anatomical barrier, the arachnoid or pia membrane. This allows for removal with a conventional laminectomy in most cases (50). The role of radiotherapy for spinal meningiomas is the same as for intracranial meningiomas. The only difference lies in the tolerance of the spinal cord to radiation which is in the order of 44 - 48 Gy at 1.8 - 2 Gy/fraction. This favours the use of stereotactic irradiation and the same techniques can be used as for intracranial lesions except for the use of the Gammaknife® which by the very nature of its construction cannot treat spinal lesions. Also the same total dose/fractionation choices and decision parameters apply as for intracranial lesions (51).

7. Conclusion

Although surgery is still regarded as the treatment of choice, radiation therapy is an effective alternative treatment, especially in the case of skull base meningiomas. In this anatomical location surgery carries a high risk of neurological morbidity, with a high chance of incomplete removal. Radiotherapy carries less morbidity than surgery. SRS, HSRT and FSRT all give equally good results. The choice of the radiation schedule is influenced by technical and radiobiological parameters.

8. References

[1] Riemenschneider M, Perry A, Reifenberger G. Histological classification and molecular genetics of meningiomas. Lancet Neurol 2006; 5:1054-54

[2] Condra KS, Buatti JM, Mendenhall WM, et al. Benign meningiomas: Primary treatment selection affects survival. Int J Radiat Oncol Biol Phys 1997;39(2):427- 436.

[3] Levine ZT, Buchanan RI, Sekhar LN, et al. Proposed grading system to predict the extent of resection and outcomes for cranial base meningiomas. Neurosurgery 1999;45(2):221–230.

[4] Newman SA. Meningiomas: A quest for the optimum therapy. J Neurosurg 1994;80:191–194.

[5] Sekhar LN, Swamy NK, Jaiswal V, et al. Surgical excision of meningiomas involving the clivus: Preoperative and intraoperative features as predictors of postoperative functional deterioration. J Neurosurg 1994;81:860–868.

[6] Kurita H, Sasaki T, Kawamoto S, et al. Role of radiosurgery in the management of cavernous sinus meningiomas. *Acta* Neurol Scand 1997;96(5):297–304.

[7] Pendl G, Schrottner O, Eustacchio S, et al. Cavernous sinus meningiomas—what is the strategy: Up-front or adjuvant gamma knife surgery? Stereotact Funct Neurosurg 1998; 70(Suppl. 1):33- 40.

[8] Taylor BW, Marcus RB, Jr, Friedman WA, et al. The meningioma controversy: Postoperative radiation therapy. Int J Radiat Oncol Biol Phys 1988;15(2):299 - 304.

[9] Goldsmith BJ, Wara WM, Wilson CB, *et al.* Postoperative irradiation for sub totally resected meningiomas. J Neurosurg 1994;80:195–201.

[10] Kondziolka D, Lunsford LD, Coffey RJ, et al. Stereotactic radiosurgery of meningiomas. J Neurosurg 1991;74:552–559.

[11] Shafron DH, Friedman WA, Buatti JM, et al. Linac radiosurgery for benign meningiomas. Int J Radiat Oncol Biol Phys 1999;43(2):321–327.

[12] Subach BR, Lunsford LD, Kondziolka D, et al. Management of petroclival meningiomas by stereotactic radiosurgery. Neurosurgery 1998;42(3):437- 445.

[13] Hakim R, Alexander E III, Loeffler JS, et al. Results of linear accelerator-based radiosurgery for intracranial meningiomas. Neurosurgery 1998;42(3):446–454

[14] Flickinger JC, Kondziolka D, Maitz AH, Lunsford LD. Gamma knife radiosurgery of imaging-diagnosed intracranial meningioma. Int J Radiat Oncol Biol Phys 56(3):801-806, 2003

[15] Schiappacasse L, Cendales R, Sallabanda K, et al. Preliminary results of helical tomotherapy in patients with complex-shape meningiomas close to the optic pathway. Med Dosim. 2011, Mar 10

[16] Schreuder AN, Jones DTL, Symons JE, *et al*. The NAC protontherapy planning system. *Strahlentherapie und Onkologie* 1999;175(Suppl.2):10 –12.

[17] Jones DTL, Schreuder AN, Symons JE, *et al*. The NAC particle therapy facilities. In: Amaldi U, Larsson B, editors.Hadron therapy in oncology. Elsevier Science B.V.; 1994.

[18] Gerweck LE, Kozin SV. Relative biological effectiveness of proton beams in clinical practice. *Radiother Oncol* 1999;50: 135–142.

[19] Fowler JF. Fractionation and therapeutic gain. The Biological basis of radiotherapy, Second Edition. Elsevier Science Publishers B.V. (Biomedical Division), 1989, pp 181-207

[20] Hall EJ. Inferring the ratio α/ß from multifraction experiments in nonclonogenic sytems. Radiobiology for the radiologists 5th edition. Lippcott, Williams & Wilkins, 2000, pp 335-348

[21] Vernimmen F.J., Slabbert JP. " Assessment of alpha/beta ratios for arteriovenous malformations, meningiomas, acoustic neuromas, and the optic chiasma" Int J Radiat Biol. 2010 Jun; 86(6):486-98

[22] Liu L, Bassano DA, Prasad SC, Hahn SS, Chung CT. The linear-quadratic model and fractionated stereotactic radiotherapy. International Journal of Radiation Oncology-Biology-Physics 57(3):827-832, 2003

[23] Hall EJ, Brenner DJ. The radiobiology of radiosurgery: Rationale for different treatment regimes for avm's and malignancies. International Journal of Radiation Oncology-Biology-Physics 25:381-385, 1993

[24] Liu D, Xu D,Zhang Z et al. Long term results of Gamma knife surgery for optic nerve sheath meningiomas. J Neurosurg. 2010 Dec, 113 Suppl: 28-33

[25] Morita A, Coffey RJ, Foote RL, et al. Risk of injury to cranialnerves after gamma knife radiosurgery for skull base meningiomas: Experience in 88 patients. J Neurosurg 1999;90(1):42–49.

[26] Verhey LJ, Smith V, Serago CF. Comparison of radiosurgery treatment modalities based on physical dose distributions. Int J Radiat Oncol Biol Phys 1998;40(2):497–505.

[27] Fowler JF. Fractionation and therapeutic gain. In: Steel GG, Adams GE, Horwich A, editors. The biological basis of radiotherapy. 2nd ed. Elsevier Publishers B.V. (Biomedical Division) 1989; p:181–207.

[28] Nedzi LA, Kooy H, Alexander E II, et al. Variables associated with the development of complications from radiosurgery of intracranial tumours. Int J Radiat Oncol Biol Phys 1991;21(3): 591–599.

[29] Smith V, Verhey L, Serago CF. Comparison of radiosurgical treatment modalities based on complication and control probabilities. Int J Radiat Oncol Biol Phys 1998;40(2):507–513.

[30] Tishler RB, Loeffler JS, Lunsford LD, *et al.* Tolerance of cranial nerves of the cavernous sinus to radiosurgery. Int J Radiat Oncol Biol Phys 1993;27(2):215–221.

[31] Leber KA, Bergloff J, Pendl G. Dose-response tolerance of the visual pathways and cranial nerves of the cavernous sinus to stereotactic radiosurgery. J Neurosurg 1988;88(1):43–50.

[32] Stiebel-Kalish H, Reich E,Gal L, et al. Visual outcome in meningiomas around anterior visual pathways treated with linear accelerator fractionated stereotactic radiotherapy. Int J Radiat Oncol Biol, Phys 2011 Feb 5.

[33] Lo SS, Cho KH, Hall WA, et al. Single dose versus fractionated stereotactic radiotherapy for meningiomas. Can J Neurol Sci, 2002 Aug; 29(3):240-8

[34] Jellinger K,Slowik F, Histological subtypes and prognostic problems in meningiomas. Journal of Neurology, Volume 208, number 4, 279-298

[35] Choi CY, Soltys SG, Gibbs IC, et al. Cyberknife stereotactic radiosurgery for treatment of atypical (WHO grade II) meningiomas. Neurosurgery, 2010 Nov;67(5):1180-8

[36] Askoxylakis V, Zabel-du Bois A, Schlegel W, et al. Patterns of failure after stereotactic radiotherapy of intracranial meningiomas. J Neurooncol, 2010 Jul; 98(3):367-72

[37] Jo K, Park HJ, Nam DH, *et al.* Treatment of atypical meningioma. J Clin Neurosci, 2010 Nov; 17(11):1362-6

[38] Rosenberg LA, Prayson RA, Lee J, et al. Long-term experience with World Health Organization grade III (malignant) meningiomas at a single institution. . Int J Radiat Oncol Biol, Phys 2009 Jun 1; 74(2):427-32

[39] Kondziolka D, Levy EL, Niranjan A, et al. Long-term outcomes after meningioma radiosurgery: Physician and patient perspectives. J Neurosurg 1999; 91(1):44 – 50.

[40] Rogers L, Gilbert M, Vogelbaum MA. Intracranial meningiomas of atypical (WHO grade II) histology. J Neuroonc. 2010 Sep; 99(3):393-405

[41] Mair R, Morris K, Scott I, et al. Radiotherapy for atypical meningiomas. J Neurosurg, 2011 Jun 24.

[42] El-Khatib M, EI Majdoub F, Hoevels M, et al. Stereotactic LINAC radiosurgery for incompletely resected or recurrent atypical and anaplastic meningiomas. Acta Neurochir (Wien), 2011 Jun 25

[43] Kano H, Takahashi JA, Katsuki T, et al. Stereotactic radiosurgery for atypical and anaplastic meningiomas. J Neurooonc 2007 Aug; 84(1):41-7

[44] Cai R, Barnett GH, Novak E, et al. Principal risk of peritumoral edema after stereotactic radiosurgery for intracranial meningioma is tumor-brain contact interface area. Neurosurgery, 2010 Mar; 66(3):513-22

[45] Conti A, Pontoriero A, Salamone C, et al. Protecting venous structures during radiosurgery for parasagittal meningiomas. NeurosurgFocus, 2009 Nov; 27(5):E11

[46] Miller RC, Foote RL, Coffey RJ, et al. Decrease in cranial nerve complications after radiosurgery for acoustic neuromas:A prospective study of dose and volume. Int J Radiat Oncol Biol Phys 1999; 43(2):305–311.

[47] Linskey ME, Flickinger JC, Lunsford LD. Cranial nerve length predicts the risk of delayed facial and trigeminal neuropathies after acoustic tumour stereotactic radiosurgery. Int J Radiat Oncol Biol Phys 1993; 25(2):227–233.

[48] Chamberlain MC, tredway TL. Adult primary intradural spinal cord tumors: a review. Curr Neurol Neurosci Rep, 2011 Jun;11(3):320-8

[49] Engelhard HH, Villano JL, Porter KR, et al. Clinical presentation, histology, and treatment in 430 patients with primary tumors of the spinal cord, spinal meninges, or cauda equine. J Neurosurg Spine. 2010 Jul; 13(1):67-77

[50] Kim CH, Chung CK. Surgical outcome of a posterior approach for large ventral intradural extramedullary spinal cord tumors. Spine (Phila Pa 1976) 2011 Apr 15; 36(8):E531-7

[51] Chang UK, Rhee CH, Youn SM, et al. Radiosurgery using the Cyberknife for benign spinal tumors: Korea Cancer Center Hospital experience. J Neuroonc. 2011 Jan; 101(1):91-9

[52] Henzel M, Gross MW, Hamm K, et al. Stereotactic radiotherapy of meningiomas; Symptomatology, acute and late toxicity. Strahlentherapie und Onkologie 2006 7:382-388

[53] Roche PH, Pellet W, Fuentes S, et al. Gamma knife radiosurgical management of petroclival meningiomas results and indications. Acta Neurochir (Wien). 2003 Oct; 145(10):883-8.

[54] Pollock BE. Stereotactic radiosurgery for intracranial meningiomas: indications and results, Neurosurg Focus. 2003 May 15;14(5) :e4.

[55] Selch MT, Ahn E, Laskari A, et al. Stereotactic radiotherapy for treatment of cavernous sinus meningiomas. Int J Radiat Oncol Biol Phys 2004 May1; 59(1):101-11.

[56] Villavicencio AT, Black PM, Shrieve DC et al. Linac radiosurgery for skull base meningiomas. Acta Neurochir (Wien). 2001 Nov; 143(11):1141-52.

[57] Vernimmen FJ, Harris JK, Wilson JA, et al. Stereotactic proton beam therapy of skull base meningiomas. Int J Radiat Oncol Biol Phys 2001 Jan 1; 49(1):99-105.

[58] Debus J., Wuendrich M, Pirzkall A, et. al. High efficacy of fractionated stereotactic radiotherapy of large base-of-skull meningiomas: long-term results. J Clin Oncol. 2001 Aug 1;19(15):3547-53.

[59] Mahadevan A, Floyd S, Wong E, et al. Clinical outcome after Hypofractionated Stereotactic Radiotherapy (HSRT) for benign skull base tumors. Comput Aided Surg. 2011, Apr6;16(3):112-20

[60] Torres RC,Frighetto L, De Salles AA, et al. Radiosurgery and stereotactic radiotherapy for intracranial meningiomas. Neurosurg Focus, 2003 May 15;14(5): e5

[61] Spiegelmann R, Cohen ZR, Nissim O, et al. Cavernous sinus meningiomas: a large Linac radiosurgery series. J Neuroonc Jun;98(2):195-202

[62] Zada G, Pagnini PG, Yu C, et al. Long-Term outcomes and patterns of tumor progression after gamma knife radiosurgery for bening meningiomas. Neurosurgery 2010 Aug;67(2):322-8

Part 2

Surgery of Meningioma

4

Neuronavigation for Intracranial Meningiomas

Erasmo Barros da Silva Jr., Jerônimo Buzetti Milano,
Luis Fernando Moura da Silva Jr., Lucas Alves Aurich and
Ricardo Ramina
Instituto de Neurologia de Curitiba
Brazil

1. Introduction

According to its location, the surgical treatment of intracranial meningioma can be of considerable challenge for the neurosurgeon. Image-guided surgery essencially provides intraoperative localization for dynamic navigation and, also, improves the surgical planning. The continuous development of neuroimaging and computated technology promotes continuous improvement of navigation techniques and applications. In the last ten years, frameless image-guided surgery, also popularized as neuronavigation, is considered standard of practice by most neurosurgical centers around the world. Its usage can range from a simple craniotomy flap localization to a deep brain tumor resection respecting tract fibers, eloquent areas and neurovascular structures. In some cases, neuronavigation may not be necessary, but, if avaliable, it should promotes a safer surgery, as it has yet to become an integral part of intracranial procedures.

Computed tomography (CT), ultrasound images and magnetic resonance imaging (MRI) have detailed 3D images to guide intracranial surgeries. The intraprocedural tracking avoids accidental complications and offers less invasive craniotomies. Delimited relevant brain structures (i.e. vessels, cranial nerves, foraminas, cerebral sulci), physiologic data such as PET or functional MRI and and tumor limits can be localized with neuronavigation either, reducing the total surgery running time.

The aplication of neuronavigation for meningioma surgery is commonly related to tumor localization. However, this concept is applied only to convexity located lesions, where craniotomy location and size are of main interest. In other types of meningioma surgery, 'find the tumor' is not a frequent problem. Neuronavigation is particularly useful in the identification of neurovascular structures near the area of interest. It also optimizes tumor debulking avoiding critical damage to close structures the neurosurgeon can´t directly see and, in large lesions, maximizes the extent of surgical removal staying within the limits of safe operability. The aim of this chapter is show how to enhance the neuronavigation usage for meningioma surgery.

2. Frame-based versus frameless image-guided surgery

Frame-based stereotactic resection was the first navigation method, rooted in cartesian coordinate system developed by Clarke and Horsley in the 1900s, and is still traditionally applied to functional procedures and deep intracranial mass biopsies. Although useful for craniotomy guidance to intracranial targets, it provided limited anatomy identification and any 3D visual guidance during a surgical procedure. Along with the disconfort in the operatory field due to the frame itself, these disadvantages limited their application to craniotomy.

The era of image-guided systems began in mid-1980s, when Roberts et al described a neuronavigation device with a sonic based digitizer. In 1987, Watanabe described a frameless intraoperative device for intracranial localization. The use of light emitting diodes (LED) on surgery was introduced in 1993, by Bucholz et al. These devices offered an extended orientation and direct visual guidance better than frame-based stereotaxy and was increasingly being adopted into routine practice through the 1990s.

With the continuous developments of image-guidance technology, the frameless image-guided surgery offers accuracy similar (although there is a non-statistically advantage) to frame-guided stereotaxy. Both methods seem to work well if performed by neurosurgeons experienced in their use. Still, neuronavigation functionality enhance neurosurgeon´s knowledge of anatomy and experience, promoting a safer and predictable procedure.

3. Pre-operative planning

To accomplish transoperative neuronavigation usage, preoperative images need to be acquired using a specific protocol and fiducials. Later, the data is transfered to a Workstation for surgery planning and then, transfered to neuronavigator. Although there are several different systems avaliable, all of them works involving the same steps.

3.1 Image acquisition

The current image-guided systems rely on preoperative imaging. These data should be obtained a few hours or one day before surgery and must respect a standard protocol of image acquisitions. The accuracy of the information obtained from the navigation system is directly related to image quality and thickness. Artifacts and motion distortion should be strongly avoided in order to prevent targer registration error. Contrast-enhanced T1-weighted 3D MRI (1.5 or 3.0 Tesla) and contrast-enhanced CT scan represents optimal choices for planning, as they assure tumor visualization. Both CT and MRI have particularities and both can be used to navigation. Image fusion between CT and MRI is particulary useful for skull base navigations, due to the correlationship of bone to soft tissues (nerves, vessels). Also, image fusion with physiologic data or vascular imaging may help avoid potential damages.

The neurosurgeon involvement starts at the acquisition, the inicial step for neuronavigation, in order to stay aware of data quality and, eventually, demands a new image acquisition.

After acquisition, images are transferred to the workstation over a local network or employing CD-ROM.

3.2 Planning in the workstation

Once in the Workstation, the data are analized and treated. Although surgical planning can be jumped, if meticulously performed, it offers neuronavigation optimization with addictional and reliable details. When multiple sequences are available, they should be fused (figure 1).

In case of anatomical landmarks registration, these structures should be determined during planning: nasion, anterior nasal spine, medial and lateral angles of the eye, tragus and ear helix can be reliable skin landmarks for usage. In case of fiducials (adhesive or skull implanted) registration, these will be clearly shown in the image data (figure 2).

Usually demonstrated as homeogenic contrast-enhanced lesions, meningiomas can be easily delimitated during surgical planning. Also, necrotic cavities, bleeding areas may be enfatized. Adjacent anatomy, such as cortical sulci and gyri, compression, adherence, and/or displacement of neurovascular structures should be analysed and, if necessary, delimitated for a 3D demonstration (figure 3 and 4).

When surgical planning is done, the worked data are transferred to the neuronavigator.

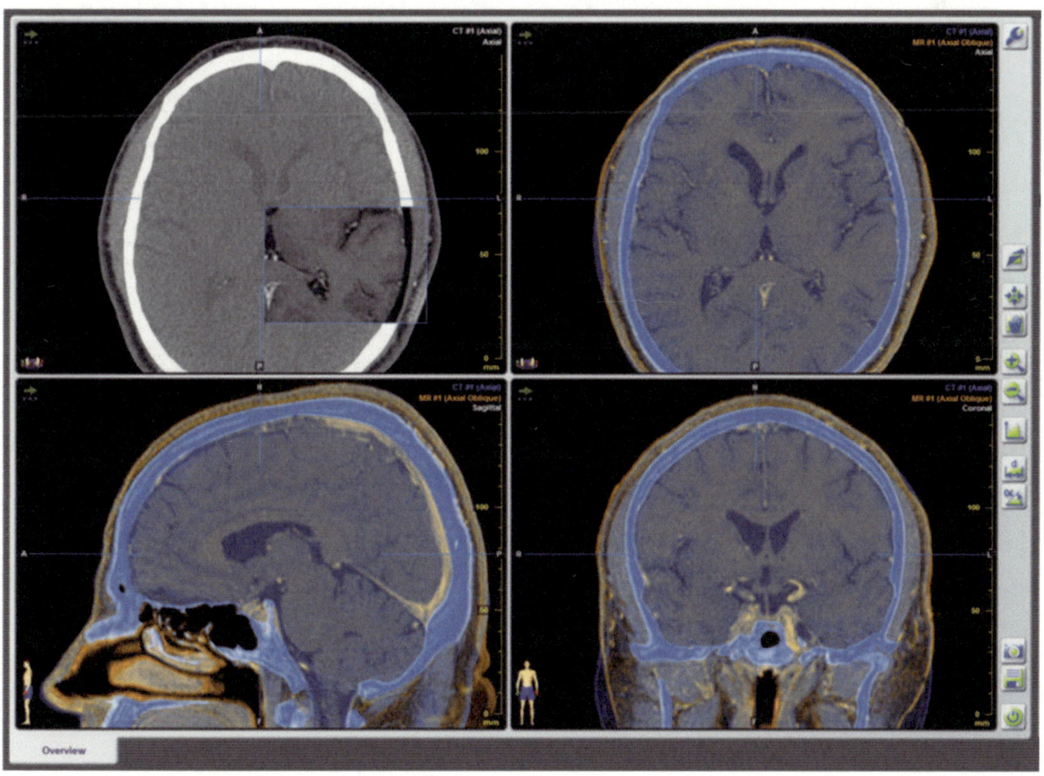

Fig. 1. CT/MRI fusion on Workstation

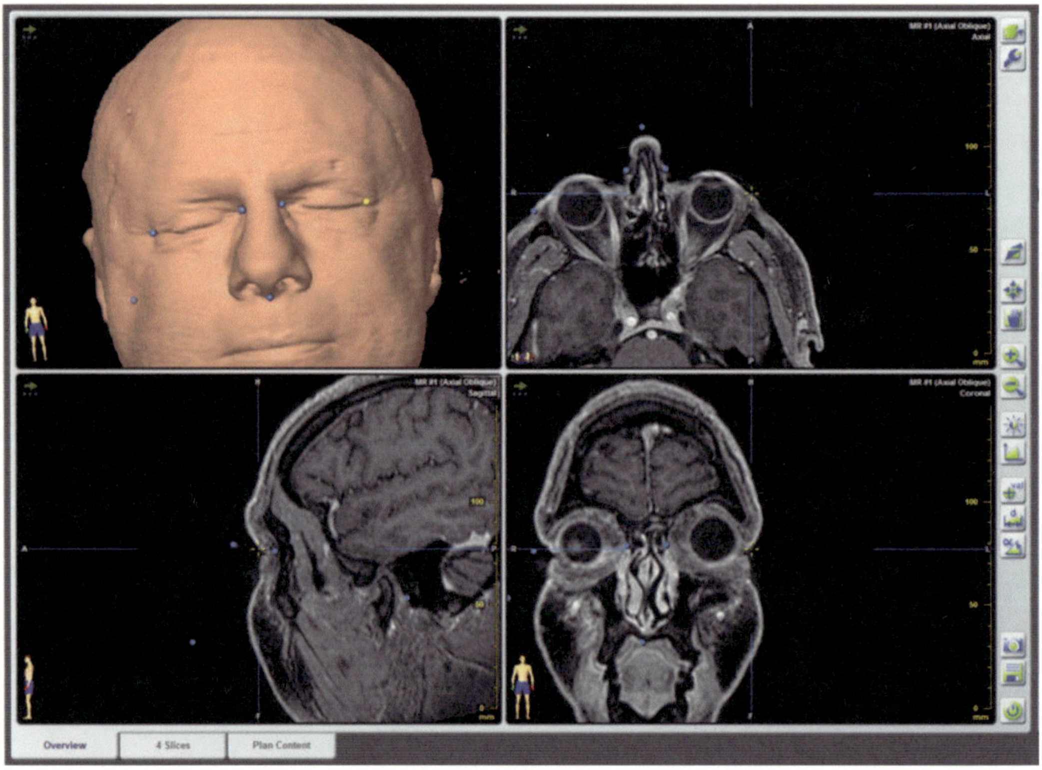

Fig. 2. Markers for registration with skin anatomical landmarks

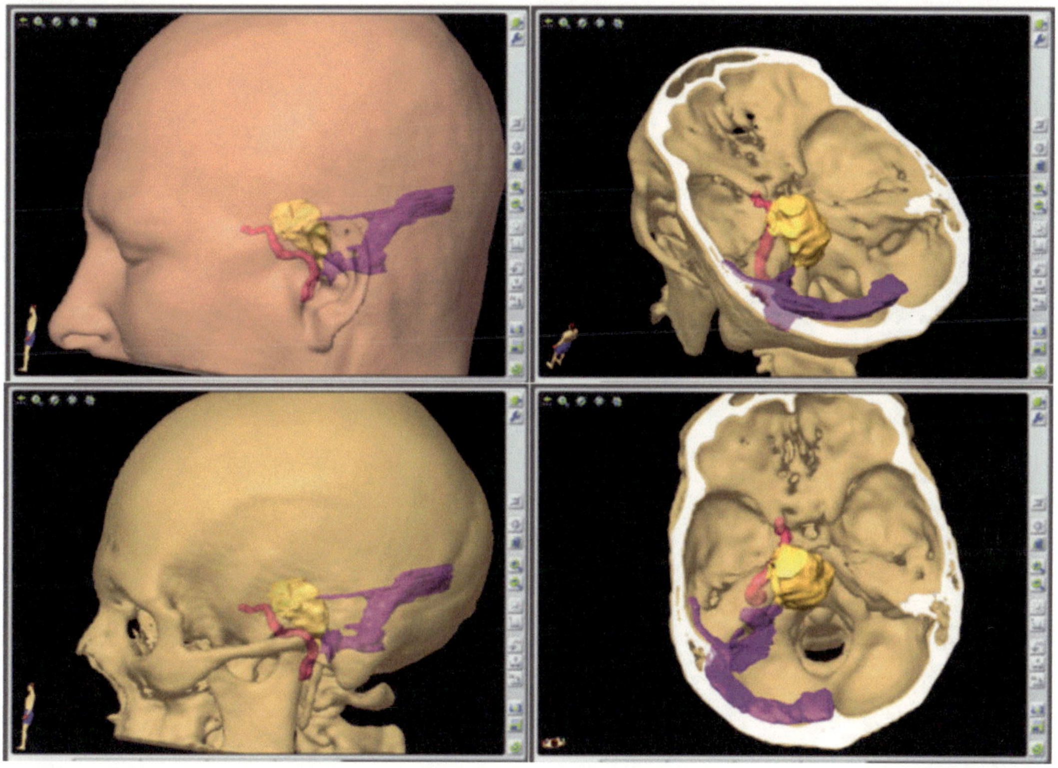

Fig. 3. Tumor (yellow) and vascular structures (purple and red) marked in the workstation for a petroclival meningioma surgery

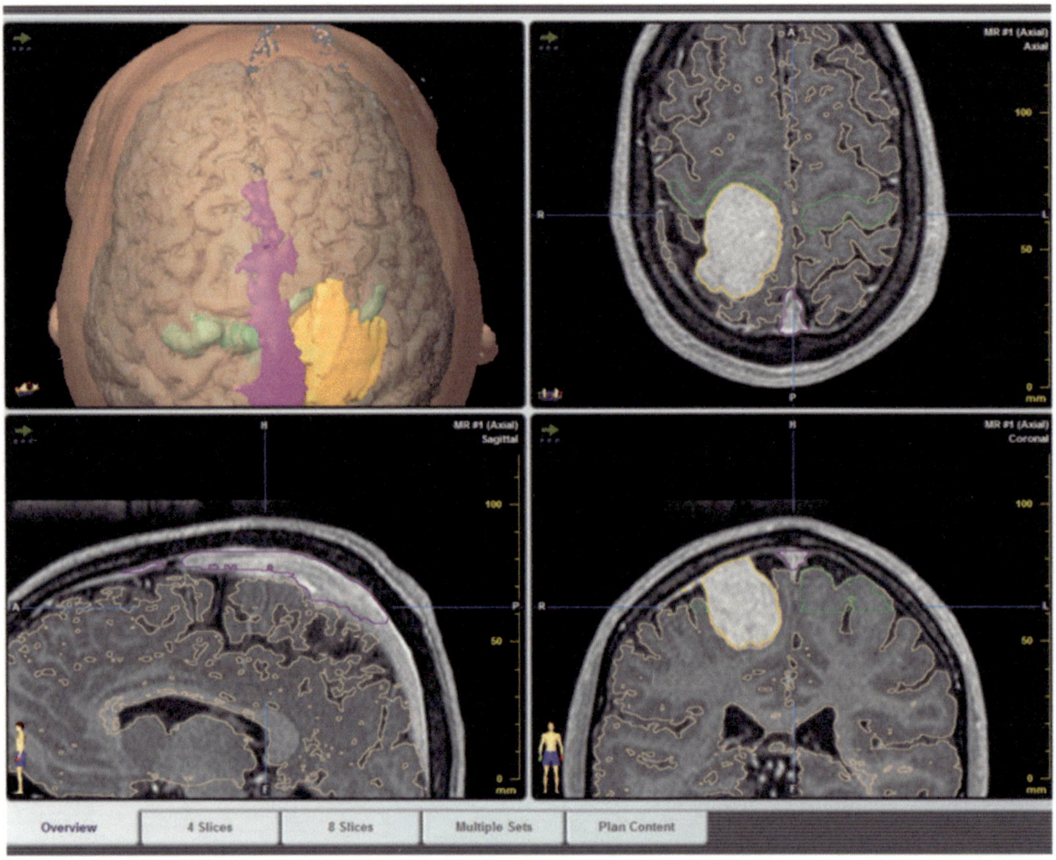

Fig. 4. A parasagital meningioma (yellow), superior sagital sinus (purple) and motor cortex (green) marked in the Workstation during surgical planning

4. Image-to-patient registration

In the operation room, after the patient's head is secured in Mayfield clamp with a reference star fixed in it and after positioning the neuronavigator camera array, patient-to-image registration is carried out (figure 5). There are three types of registration methods for navigation which should be designated according to the target area/tumor location. In some cases, as usually occurs in posterior fossa approachs, there is a common concept of major accuracy flaw due to image distortion and registration fiducials/anatomical landmarks too far from area of interest. However, these pitfalls may be avoided with a few considerations.

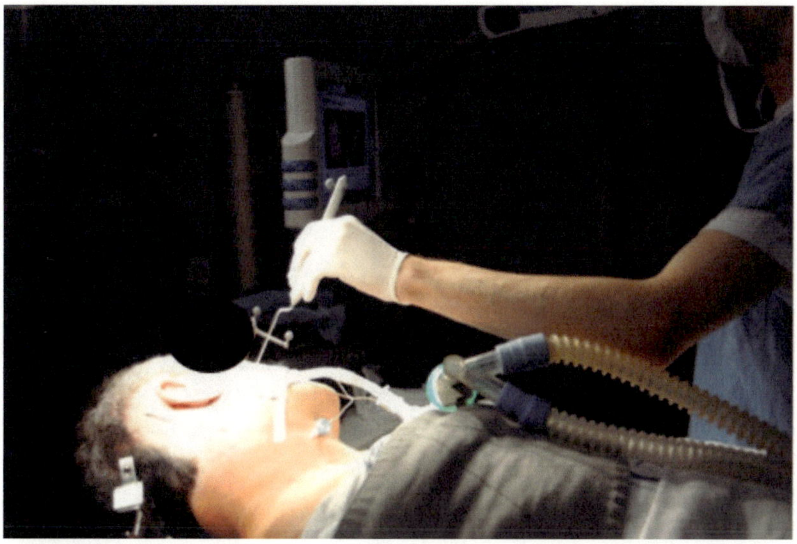

Fig. 5. Patient registration

Fiducials (figure 6 and 7) is the most frequently method of registration. It consists in the use of 4-8 (usually 6) fiducials placed in predetermined positions (usually near the area of interest) upon patient's scalp and imaging with standardised protocols. These fiducials may be skull implanted, which is invasive 'gold standard', with an accuracy flaw below 2 mm; or adhesive to the skin, and carried out the day before surgery or sometimes immediately prior to surgery. Consequently, fiducials usage demands time, delaying surgery, and adds extra costs.

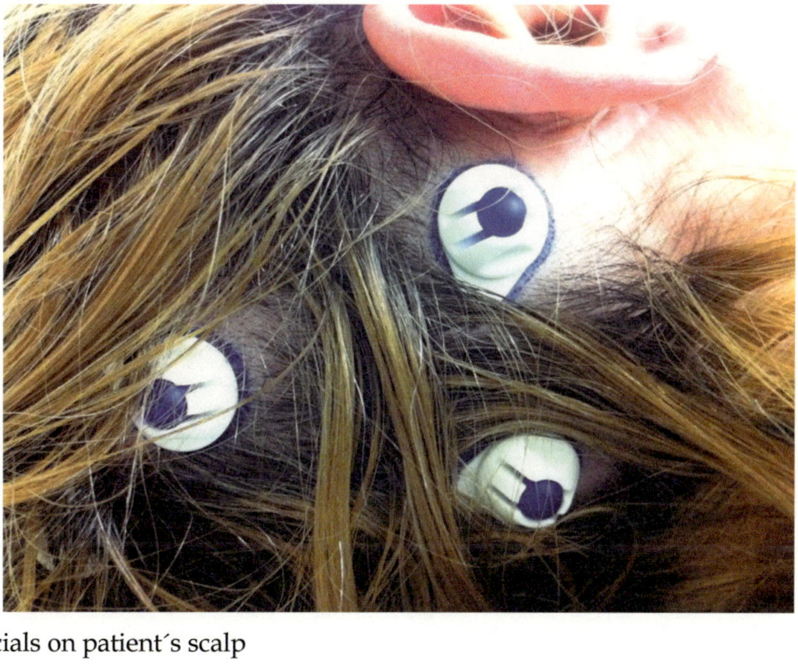

Fig. 6. Fiducials on patient´s scalp

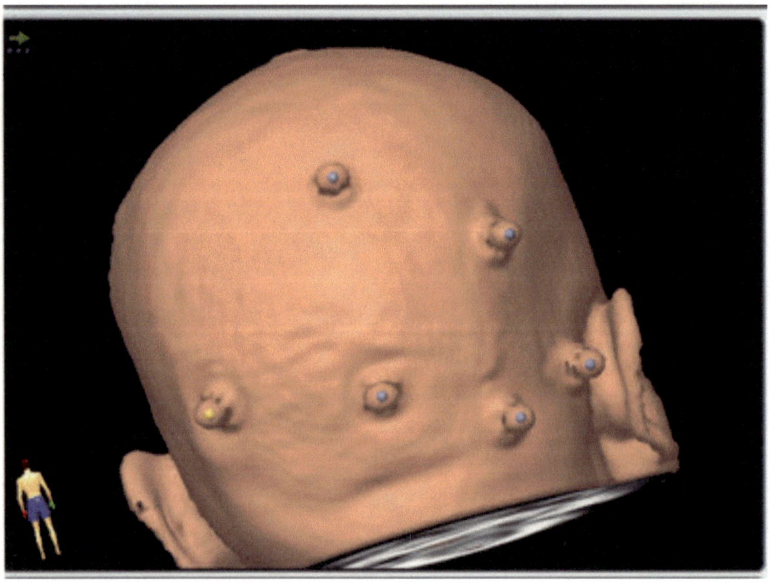

Fig. 7. Fiducials on patient´s scalp in workstation

Skin surface based registration (figure 8) consists of a LASER pointer registration over patient´s forehead, nose and around eyes. These method usually provides a reliable accuracy for craniofacial or anterior skull base surgery. Due to image distortion, there´s an increasingly accuracy flaw posterior to coronal suture/ear. Although limited usage, it doesn´t demands a preparation during surgical planning and may be complemented with anatomical landmarks acquisition to enhance the registration.

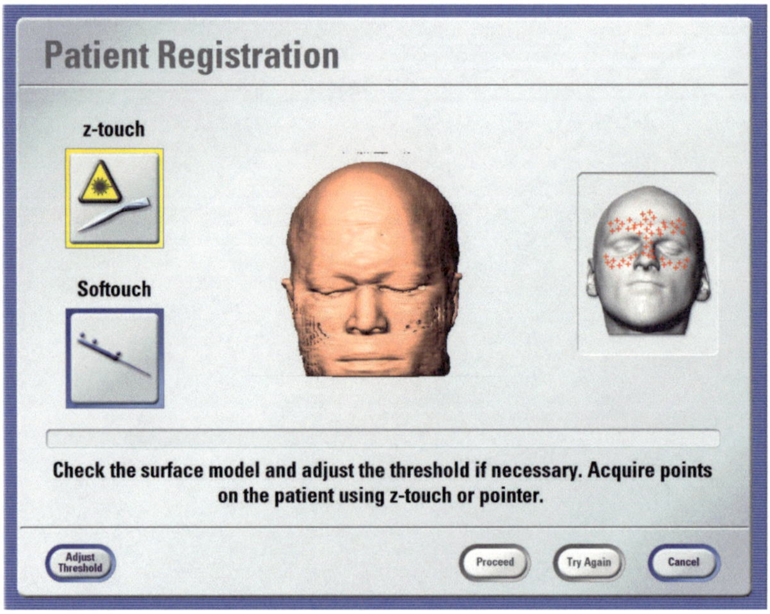

Fig. 8. Surface matching registration (navigator screen)

Registration with anatomical landmarks consists in the use of anatomical landmarks instead of fiducial markers. In patients face, these landmarks can be nasion, anterior nasal spine, medial and lateral angles of the eyes and other points carefully choosen in order to avoid distortion or too mobile areas . It may be the most operator-dependent method of registration and still the possibility of registration using bone instead of skin anatomical landmarks. Foramina, angles and sutures on bone anatomy (figure 9 and 10) usually offers reliable landmarks for registration and are performed after skin incision. This method is often used during navigation in spinal procedures. Once the necessary landmarks are exposed on the operatory field, registration can be and provides a more logical consistency in anatomical landmarks usage. As these points are closer to the area of interest than any skin fiducials, it favors the registration to a better accuracy for targets in deep structures.

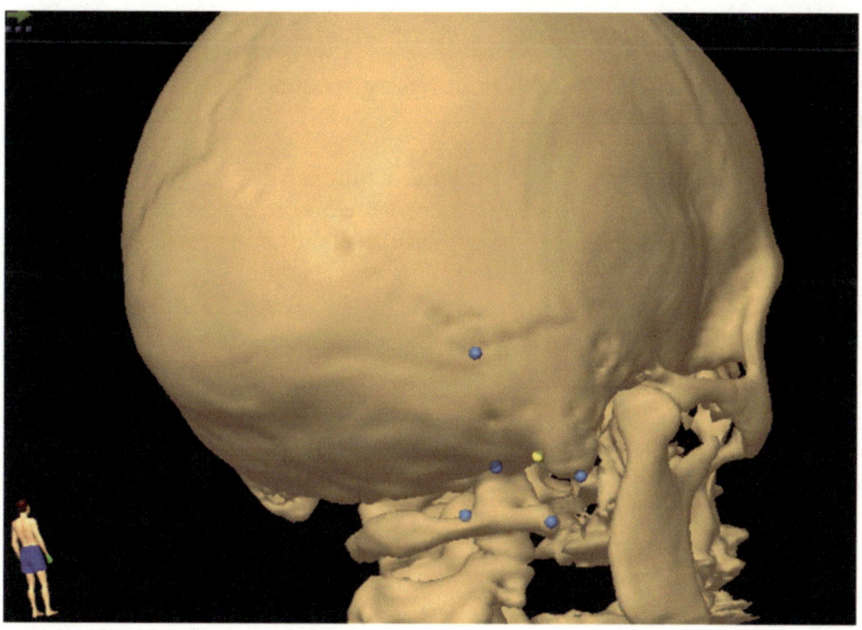

Fig. 9. Anatomical landmarks for intraoperative registration - lateral craniocervical approach

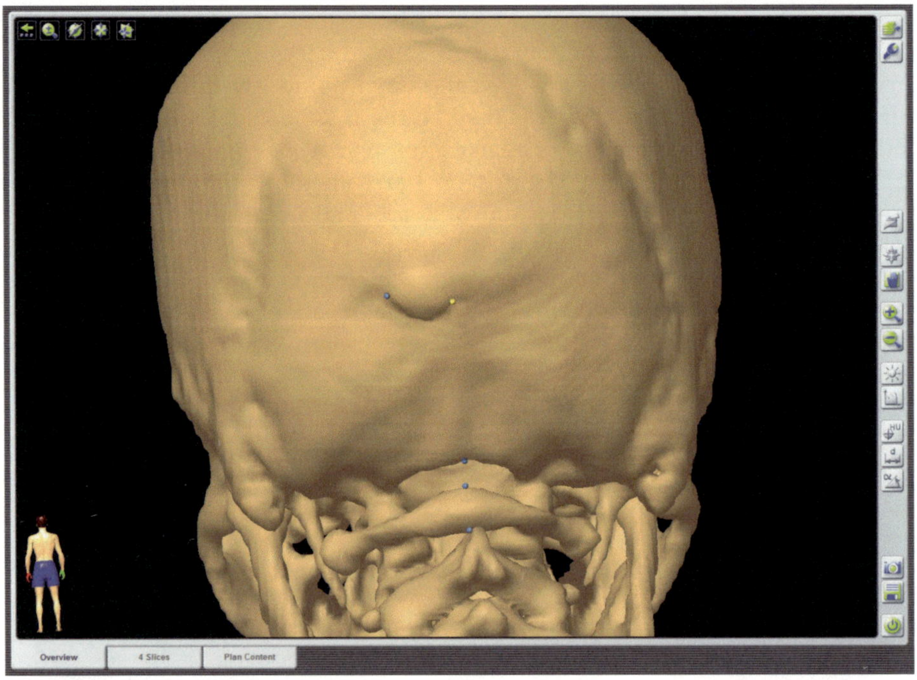

Fig. 10. Anatomical landmarks for intraoperative registration - suboccipital midline approach

For most surgeries, an accuracy flaw around 2-4 mm can be accepted, specially for large target areas. The target registration error may vary according to the utilized navigation system, but data imaging and its correlation with the landmarks during registration consist decisive factors to neuronavigation success. Nonetheless, the surgeon should be familiar with the limitations and potential sources of error in all steps involved neuronavigation before intraoperative tracking.

Some possible erros for accuracy flaw involves shifting. First, the reference star, which should be well-attached to the head fixer to avoid any kind of deslocation; second, patient´s head deslocation in the Mayfield clamp; and, finally, brain-shift, which isn´t accidental and can be, on most cases, a predictable event.

Brain-shifting may be avoided with new image data (ultrasound, CT or MRI) acquisition intraoperatively, when available. However, the distortion in meningioma surgery usually is minimal and avoidable in most cases, specially when the navigation focus lies on a well-centered minimal invasive craniotomy. In skull base meningioma surgery, this distortion still avoidable due to the extensive bone work.

5. Intra-operative tracking based on tumor location

Meningioma surgery may involve different challenges for the surgeon, according to its size, location, relationship and adherence with brain and neurovascular scructures. It may vary from a simple small frontal convexity meningioma resection to a large petroclival tumor surgery involving cranial nerves and compressing brainstem from posterior to middle fossa.

Discuss the neuronavigation utility for meningioma surgery must be focused based on tumor location. According to each case, there are ways to optimize its usage beyond the misunderstood 'find the tumor' concept.

5.1 Convexity meningiomas

For most neurosurgical centers, convexity meningiomas probably is the standard for neuronavigation usage in meningioma surgery due to its urgency in place the craniotomy in the right place.

Contrast enhanced images are the preferred modality for both CT scan and MRI , since the objective is 'see' the lesion. During surgical planning, a surgical trajectory should be defined determining the size and location for craniotomy. The 3D reconstrution allows an optimal view and avoids mistakes. For image-to-patient registration, surface matching may be an useful method for tumors anterior to coronal suture, but adhesive fiducials to the scalp still the safest choice.

After skin incision, the image-guided craniotomy should be at least a 2cm larger than the maximum diameter of tumor´s dural base. It will provide an better area to tumor removal and duroplasty (figure 8).

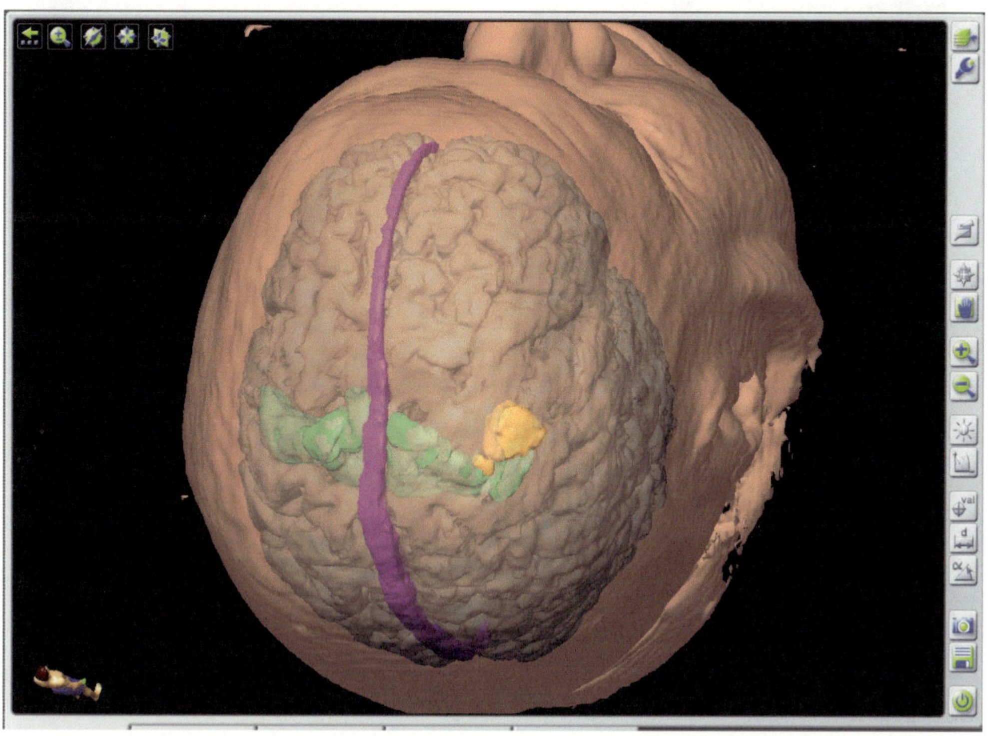

Fig. 11. Convexity meningioma on Workstation: tumor (yellow), superior sagital sinus (purple) and motor cortex (green)

Brain-shifting usually is a minor treat for neuronavigation in these cases because the optimal place for craniotomy is determined before. Still, the tumor lies attached to dural tail and bone. Venous anatomy, specially those underlying the dura, may be understood with neuronavigation, providing an adequate dural opening avoiding accidental bleeding.

5.2 Parasagital and falcine meningiomas

Although the craniotomy for parasagital/falcine meningiomas can be planned considering only tumor relationship with the superior sagital sinus, neuronavigation is important to display underlying venous anatomy and the midline. The use of MRI provides the necessary data for planning, where the relevant structures can be marked (figure 12). Vascular studies should always be available for addicional information and, eventually, data fusion.

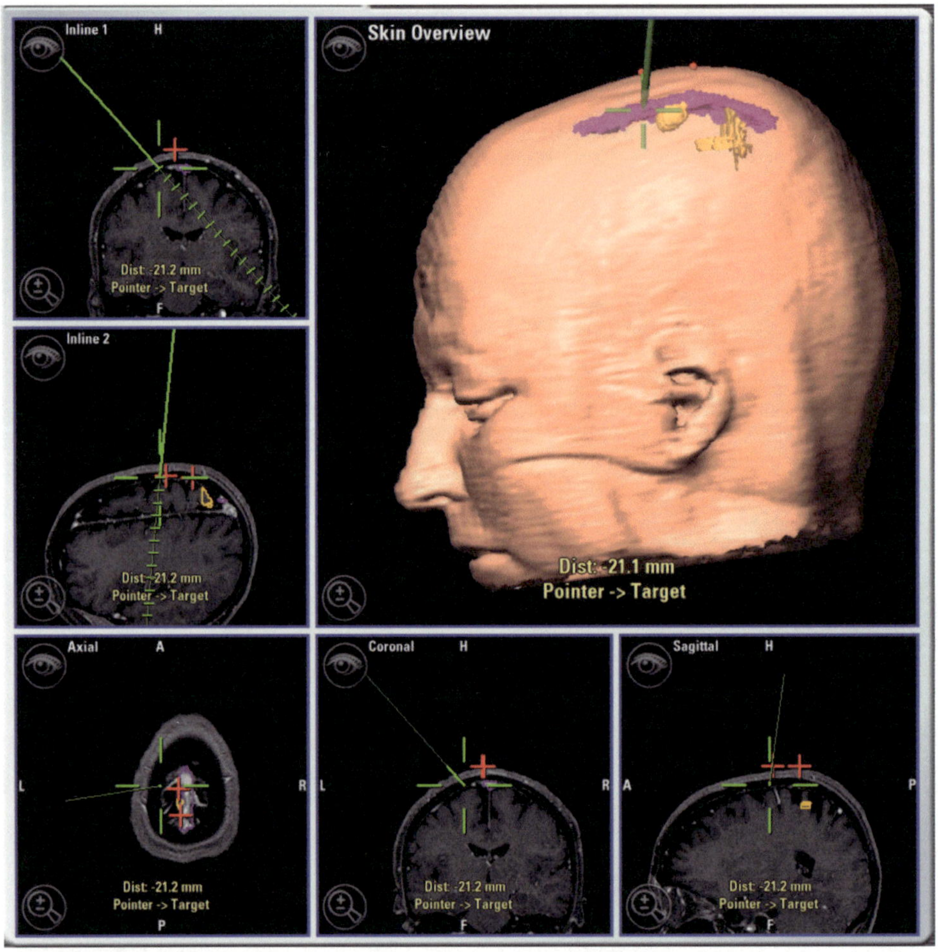

Fig. 12. Parasagital meningioma navigation during craniotomy placement

The method of registration is similar to convexity meningiomas, where fiducials are the preferred and surface matching reliable only for lesions in the anterior 1/3 of the superior sagital sinus and falx.

For falcine tumor, the neuronavigation should provide a safe surgical corridor between draining veins and midline. The brain-shifting is still a rare problem, as these tumors are tethered to fixed structures such as superior sagital sinus and falx. Once more, draining veins and major arterial branches can be predicted with neuronavigation assistance. For large tumors, functional MRI may promote a better understanding of the distorted cerebral eloquent anatomy to avoid post-operative deficits.

5.3 Tentorial meningiomas

For tentorial meningiomas surgery, the neuronavigation shoud provides important information in the understanding of venous anatomy. Although the approach, both supra and infratentorial, doesn´t depends to neuronavigation, the exactly midline localization provided by the system aids to deal with the dural sinuses. The transverse sinuses location should be located either, avoiding a major bleeding risk during craniotomy (figure 13).

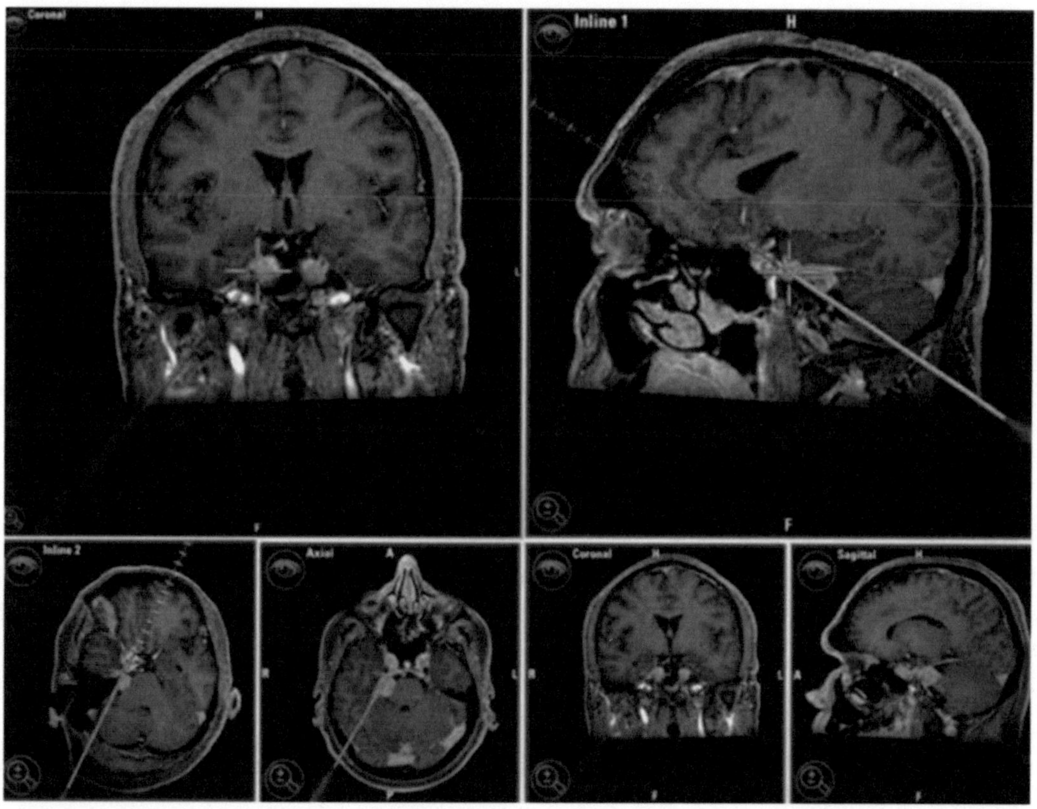

Fig. 13. Tentorial meningioma navigation

Fiducial markers are the best choice for registration, and they should be placed near the area of interest and dural sinuses.

Location of the vein of Labbe can be identified with navigation to avoid damage during dural opening, for supratentorial lesions. Also, distorted deep venous drainage can be identified when the surgeon is working near the midline.

5.4 Olfatory groove and suprasellar meningiomas

For skull base navigation, CT/MRI fusion should always be considered. There will be a special reliability in neuronavigation, since the surgeon will aim bone and fixed structures. In anterior fossa meningiomas surgery, neuronavigation isn´t necessary for craniotomy, as they usually demand a frontolateral approach.

Surface matching can be a reliable method for registration in anterior fossa meningioma surgery. During surgery, the neuronavigation can be used before dural opening to frontal sinus identification, and after in order to determine tumor relationship with midline, oftatory groove, optic nerves and internal carotid arteries. The relevant anatomy may be marked in surgical planning. Also, the neuronavigation should aid to show the position during tumor debulking, specially when approaching posterior structures such as infundibulum.

5.5 Sphenoid wing and cavernous sinus meningiomas

Sphenoid wing and cavernous sinus meningiomas can be accessed using a pterional approach and its variants without the need for neuronavigation. However, it can provide valuable intraoperative information during tumor debulking as the location of vascular structures distorted by the tumor. The mesial structures, including cavernous sinus, can be identified without accuracy loss due to brain-shifting, as these structures remain attached to skull base.

Fiducial markers and surface matching are good choices for registration, as well, anatomical landmarks, especially if mixing skin landmarks (before skin incision) and bone landmarks (after skin incision) such as key hole and zygomatic arch.

Neurophysiologic monitoring is always an valiable tool to help predict cranial nerves location and, with neuronavigation support for spatial orientation, reduces post-operative deficits.

5.6 Petroclival and jugular forame meningiomas

The neuronavigation usage for posterior fossa tumors can be divided in an extra-dural application, specially during the craniotomy, helping determine dural sinuses location, and an intra-dural application, aiding tumor debulking and avoiding inadvertent neurovascular damage. CT/MRI fusion is essencial for neuronavigation in these cases.

The registration technique may vary to fiducial markers and, according to the approach, anatomical landmarks. There is a special challenge for posterior fossa registration due to distortion and accuracy loss and it may be avoided with registration hints. For a retrosigmoid craniotomy, skin anatomical landmarks can provide a reliable registration. For craniocervical lateral approachs and suboccipital midline approachs, there will be enough bone anatomical landmarks (such as inion, foramen magnun borders, atlas arch, digastric incisure, mastoid tip) to use for registration, with the advantage of more proximity from the area of interest and, consequently, a minor target registration error (figure 14). Although faster than fiducial markers, anatomical landmarks registration demands more familiarity and experience with the method than other methods of registration.

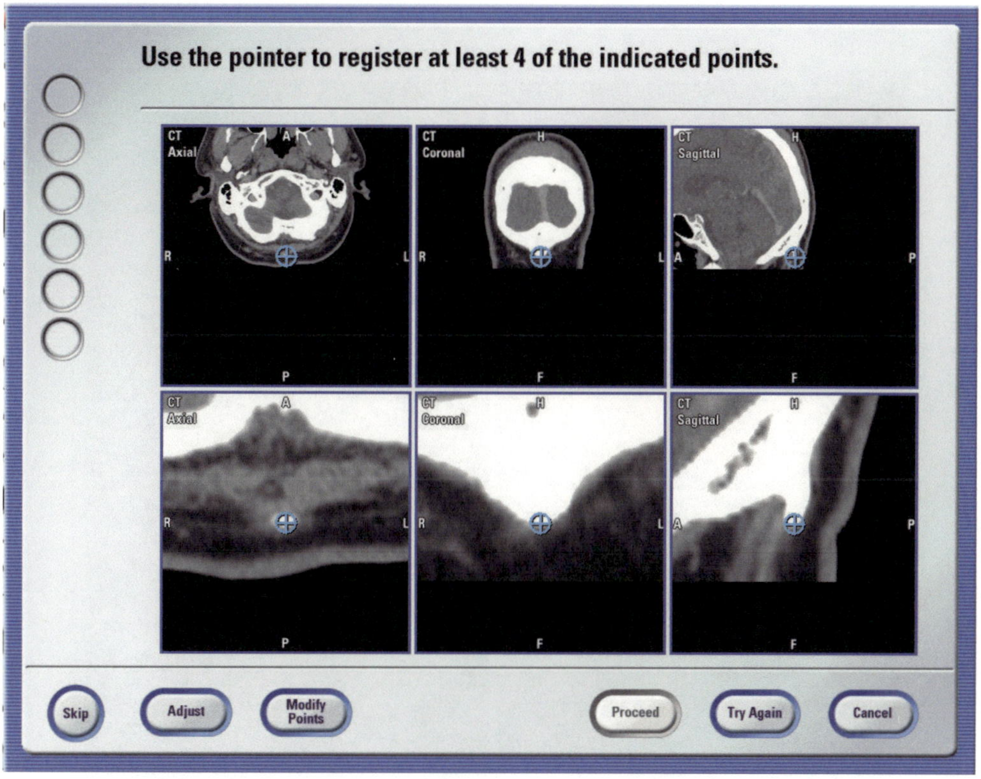

Fig. 14. Intra-operative registration with anatomical landmarks on bone anatomy (Inion)

The transverse and sigmoid sinuses should be marked in surgical planning to optimal positioning of lateral craniotomies (figure 15). In midline approaches, the torculla as well the transverse sinuses are marked delimiting the supratentorial from infratentorial dura. The intradural usage of neuronavigation may be suceptible to accuracy error if the registration wasn´t skillfully performed. Tumor limits and foramina can be identified with neuronavigation support. Although cranial nerves are hard to mark in the surgical planning, vessels position can be predicted using to same tool. It is specially important in determine the location of basilar and vertebral arteries, hidden by the tumor. Still, the neuronavigation is a reliable tool for surgeon´s orientation through midline when debulking large tumors with brainstem displacement.

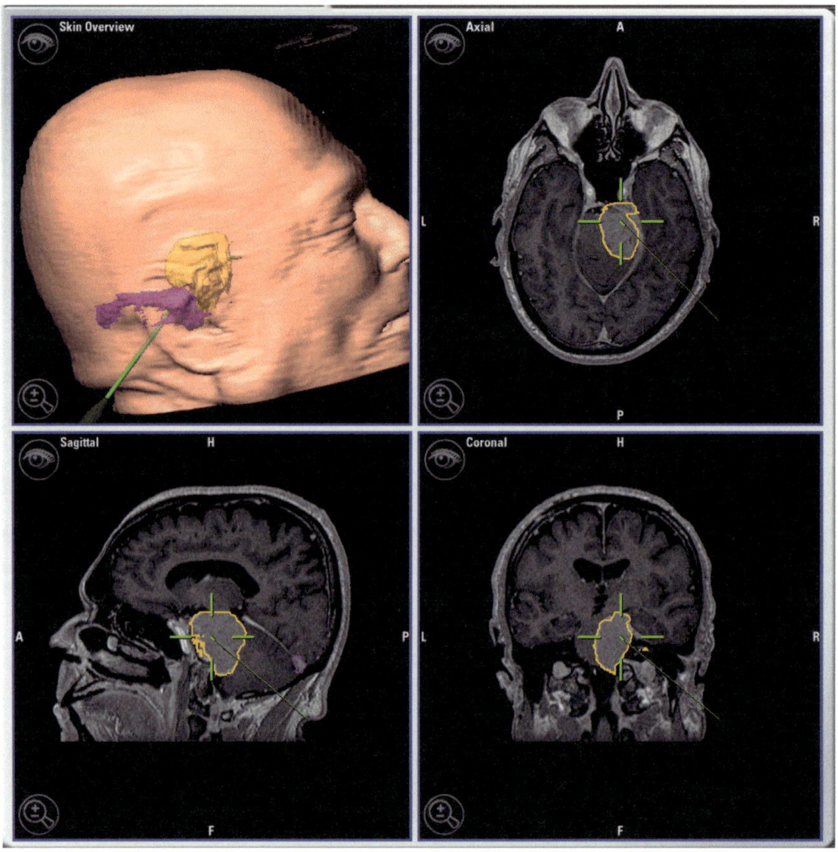

Fig. 15. Navigation for a petroclival meningioma: tumor (yellow) and transverse-sigmoid sinuses (purple)

In case of craniocervical approachs, the neuronavigation can aid to identify the relevant anatomy of the neck dissection, such as carotid and vertebral arteries (figure 16).

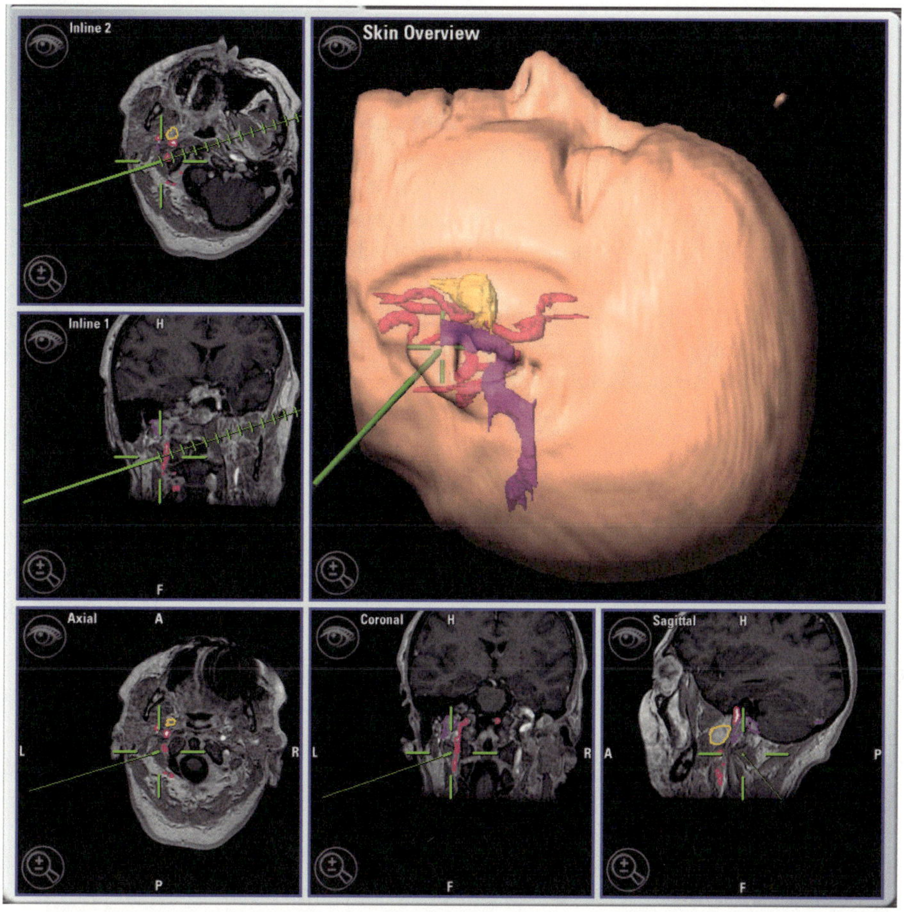

Fig. 16. Navigation for a jugular forame meningioma: tumor (yellow), transverse-sigmoid sinuses and jugular bulb (purple) and posterior arterial circulation (red)

6. Final considerations: Future applications of image-guided surgery for intracranial meningiomas

Image guided surgical technology plays a significant role in contemporary neurosurgery that doesn´t exclude the neurosurgeon´s anatomy knowledge and personal experience. It is a tool designed to aggregate more information to the surgery, specially with the preoperative planning. It also provides continuous new possibilities and perspectives for surgical treatments, as neuroimaging is improving through the years. The main goal for neuronavigation in meningioma surgery stands in optimal craniotomies, less dural sinuses damage and safer tumor removal. The method don´t aims to turn the surgery 'easier', but 'safer', and in reliable ways.

7. References

Barnett GH, Steiner CP, Weisenberger J. Intracranial meningioma resection using frameless stereotaxy. *J Image Guid Surg.* 1(1):46-52, 1995.

Benardete EA, Leonard MA, Weiner HL: Comparison of Frameless Stereotactic Systems: Accuracy, Precision, and Applications. *Neurosurgery* 49:1409-1015, 2001.

da Silva EB Jr, Leal AG, Milano JB, da Silva LF Jr, Clemente RS, Ramina R: Image-guided surgical planning using anatomical landmarks in the retrosigmoid approach. *Acta Neurochir (Wien)* 152:905-910, 2010.

Esquia-Medina G, Nguyen Y, Mazalaigue S, Vellin JF, Lombard B, Kalamarides M, Ferrary E, Sterkers O. Use of anatomic or invasive markers in association with skin surface registration in image-guided surgery of the temporal bone. *Acta Otolaryngol.* 2009 Jan 19:1-6.

Gharabaghi A, Rosahl SK, Feigl GC, Liebig T, Mirzayan JM, Heckl S, Shahidi R, Tatagiba M, Samii M. Image-guided lateral suboccipital approach: part 1-individualized landmarks for surgical planning. *Neurosurgery.* 62(3 Suppl 1):18-22; discussion 22-3, 2008.

Gharabaghi A, Rosahl SK, Feigl GC, Safavi-Abbasi S, Mirzayan JM, Heckl S, Shahidi R, Tatagiba M, Samii M. Image-guided lateral suboccipital approach: part 2-impact on complication rates and operation times. *Neurosurgery.* 2008 Mar;62(3 Suppl 1):24-9; discussion 29.

Gharabaghi A, Rosahl SK, Feigl GC, Samii A, Liebig T, Heckl S et al. Surgical planning for retrosigmoid craniotomies improved by 3D computed tomography venography. *Eur J Surg Oncol* 34(2):227-31, 2008.

Greenfield JP, Cobb WS, Tsouris AJ, Schwartz TH. Stereotactic minimally invasive tubular retractor system for deep brain lesions. *Neurosurgery.* 2008 Oct;63(4 Suppl 2):334-9; discussion 339-40.

Hill DLG, Hawkes DJ, Crossman JE, Gleeson MJ, Cox TCS, Bracey EECML et al. Registration of MR and CT images for skull base surgery using point-like anatomical features. *Br J Radiol* 64(767): 1030-35, 1991.

Holly LT, Foley KT: Intraoperative spinal navigation. *Spine.* 28:54-61, 2003

Keskil S, Bademci G, Goksel M. Tracing the dural tail with image-guided surgery. *Minim Invasive Neurosurg.* 2006 Dec;49(6):357-8.

Low D, Lee CK, Dip LL, Ng WH, Ang BT, Ng I. Augmented reality neurosurgical planning and navigation for surgical excision of parasagittal, falcine and convexity meningiomas. *Br J Neurosurg* 24(1):69-74, 2010.

Marmulla R, Mühling J, Wirtz CR, Hassfeld S. High-resolution laser surface scanning for patient registration in cranial computer-assisted surgery. *Minim Invasive Neurosurg.* 2004 Apr;47(2):72-8.

Mascott CR, Sol JC, Bousquet P, Lagarrigue J, Lazorthes Y, Lauwers-Cances V. Quantification of true in vivo (application) accuracy in cranial image-guided surgery: influence of mode of patient registration. *Neurosurgery.* 2006 Jul;59(1 Suppl 1):ONS146-56.

Maurer CR, Rohlfing T, Dean D, West JB, Rueckert D, Mori K, et al : *Sources of error in image registration for cranial image-guided neurosurgery,* in Germano IM (ed): Advanced Techniques in Image-Guided Brain and Spine Surgery. New York: Thieme, 2002, pp 10–36.

Morokoff AP, Zauberman J, Black PM. Surgery for convexity meningiomas. *Neurosurgery* 2008;63(3):427-33, 2008.

Nakao N, Nakai K, Itakura T: Updating of neuronavigation based on images intraoperatively acquired with a mobile computerized tomographic scanner: technical note. *Minim Invasive Neurosurg* 46:117-120, 2003

Nimsky C, Ganslandt O, Cerny S, Hastreiter P, Greiner G, Fahlbusch R: Quantification of, visualization of, and compensation for brain shift using intraoperative magnetic resonance imaging. *Neurosurgery* 47:1070-1079, 2000.

Nimsky C, von Keller B, Schlaffer S, Kuhnt D, Weigel D, Ganslandt O, et al: Updating navigation with intraoperative image data. *Top Magn Reson Imaging* 19:197-204, 2009.

Pfisterer WK, Papadopoulos S, Drumm DA, Smith K, Preul MC. Fiducial versus nonfiducial neuronavigation registration assessment and considerations of accuracy. *Neurosurgery* 62(3):201-7, 2008.

Omay SB, Barnett GH. Surgical navigation for meningioma surgery. *J Neurooncol* 99(3):357-64, 2010.

Paleologos TS, Wadley JP, Kitchen ND, Thomas DG. Clinical utility and cost-effectiveness of interactive image-guided craniotomy: clinical comparison between conventional and image-guided meningioma surgery. *Neurosurgery*. 47(1):40-7; discussion 47-8 (2000).

Ramina R, Neto MC, Fernandes YB, Ramina KLF: *Meningiomas do Seio Cavernoso*, in Aguiar PHP, Ramina R, Veiga JCE, Tella Jr O (Eds): Meningiomas - diagnóstico e tratamento clínico e cirúrgico: aspectos atuais. Rio de Janeiro: Revinter, 2006, pp 161-170.

Ramina R, Neto MC, Fernandes YB, Maniglia JJ, Clemente R: *Meningiomas do Forame Magno*, in Aguiar PHP, Ramina R, Veiga JCE, Tella Jr O (Eds): Meningiomas - diagnóstico e tratamento clínico e cirúrgico: aspectos atuais. Rio de Janeiro: Revinter, 2006, pp 185-191.

Reinacher PC, van Velthoven V. Intraoperative ultrasound imaging: practical applicability as a real-time navigation system. *Acta Neurochir* 85:89-93, 2003.

Roberts DW, Strohbehn JW, Hatch JF, Murray W, Kettenberger H. A frameless stereotaxic integration of computerized tomographic imaging and the operating microscope. *J Neurosurg* 65:545-9, 1986.

Rosahl SK, Shahidi R: *The Virtual Operating Field – How Image Guidance can Become Integral to Microneurosurgery*, in Ramina R, Aguiar PHP, Tatagiba M(Eds): Samii's Essentials in Neurosurgery. Berlim: Springer, 2008, pp 11-20.

Samset E, Høgetveit JO, Cate GT, Hirschberg H: Integrated neuronavigation system with intraoperative image updating. *Minim Invasive Neurosurg*. 48:73-76, 2005

Schulder M, Sernas TJ, Carmel PW. Cranial surgery and navigation with a compact intraoperative MRI system. *Acta Neurochir* 85:79-86, 2003.

Solheim O, Selbekk T, Lindseth F, Unsgård G. Navigated resection of giant intracranial meningiomas based on intraoperative 3D ultrasound. *Acta Neurochir (Wien)*. 151(9):1143-51, 2009.

Wadley J, Dorward N, Kitchen N, Thomas D. Pre-operative planning and intra-operative guidance in modern neurosurgery: a review of 300 cases. *Ann R Coll Surg Engl*. 81(4):217-25, 1999.

Wang MN, Song ZJ. Properties of the target registration error for surface matching in neuronavigation. *Comput Aided Surg*. 16(4):161-9. 2011.

Westendorff C, Kaminsky J, Ernemann U, Reinert S, Hoffmann J. Image-guided sphenoid wing meningioma resection and simultaneous computer-assisted cranio-orbital reconstruction: technical case report. *Neurosurgery.* 60(2):ONSE173-4; discussion ONSE174, 2007.

Wirtz CR, Bonsanto MM, Knauth M, Tronnier VM, Albert FK, Staubert A, et al: Intraoperative magnetic resonance imaging to update interactive navigation in neurosurgery: method and preliminary experience. *Comput Aided Surg.* 2:172-179, 1997

Wolfsberger S, Rössler K, Regatschnig R, Ungersböck K. Anatomical landmarks for image registration in frameless stereotactic neuronavigation. *Neurosurg Rev* 25:68-72, 2002.

5

Surgical Management of Skull Base Meningiomas – An Overview

Bernhard R. Fischer and Benjamin Brokinkel
Department of Neurosurgery, University Hospital of Münster
Germany

1. Introduction

Meningiomas as extra axial tumours, developing from arachnoid cap cells may occur from all dural structures, cranial and spinal and rarely outside of these structures (Whittle et al. 2004). The skull base is an area with multiple neural structures as well as brain supplying adjacent arteries and veins. Meningiomas, growing on or within the skull can thus be very challenging for the neurosurgeon. In consequence, complete tumour removal without neural impairment is not always possible (Seifert 2010; Yasargil 1980) and surgery in this area, especially in petro-clival meningiomas, hazardous. Advances in microsurgical technique, development of new approaches and advancement of adjuvant therapies allow for reducing or removing meningiomas as well as a sufficient control of residual or recurrent tumours.

2. Epidemiology

Meningioma is considered the most primary intracranial neoplasm, representing 14.3-19.0% of all intracranial tumours. Hence, estimated prevalence is approximately 100/100.000 with an age adjusted, sex dependent incidence rate of 8.4 and 3.6/100.000 a year.

According to the current WHO classification, the vast majority of these tumours are classified as grade I (aka benign meningioma, approximately 80-90%). With a distinct increase of recurrence and mortality, about 4.7 up to 20% of meningiomas are characterized as grade II (aka atypical) meningioma, while grade III (aka anaplastic) tumours occur in 1.0-2.8% of all meningiomas (Louis et al. 2007). Although meningioma appears presumably in all groups of age with even infants being affected, incidence peaks markedly in the fourth and sixth decade (Chohan et al. 2011; Rockhill et al. 2007). Sex distribution depicts female pre-dominace among all groups of age with a distinct apex of almost 2:1 in the 30s and 40s (Rockhill et al. 2007; Whittle et al. 2004; Wiemels et al. 2010).

3. Etiology

Although most meningiomas occur presumably spontaneously and therefore independently of neither endogenous nor exogenous factors, high and low-dose ionizing cranial radiation could be shown to induce especially meningiomas of higher grades of malignancy (Louis et al. 2007; Wiemels et al. 2010). Pronounced female predominance among patients in the fertile decades and various expression of progesterone, estrogen and androgen receptors suggest impact of sex hormones on tumour genesis and growth. Subsequently, a relation between the administration of oral contraceptives/ exogenous hormones (hormone replacement therapy, HRT) and an increased risk of meningioma development was observed (Michaud et al. 2010). Hence, these observations remain controversial and the role of sex hormones in tumour genesis needs to be determined in further analyses.

About 20% of meningiomas in adults occur in patients suffering from neurofibromatosis type 1 (Wiemels et al. 2010).

4. Locations

Approximately one third of meningiomas are classified as typical skull base meningioma, subsuming tumours arising from the arachnoids of the olfactory groove (< 10%), the tuberculum sellae (12.8%), the foramen magnum (<4%) and the sphenoid ridge (17%). The least includes meningiomas arising from either the medial, clinoidal, alar or outer, temporal/pterional portion of the sphenoid ridge (30.1%, 6.9% and 16% of all meningiomas involving the sphenoid ridge, respectively) (Honig et al. 2010; Mendenhall et al. 2004; Condra et al. 1997; Rockhill et al. 2007).

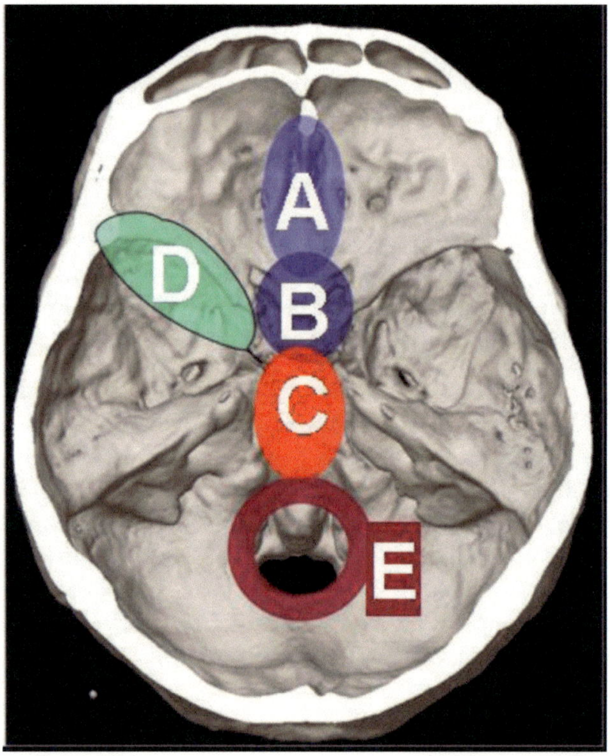

Fig. 1. Computed tomography of the scull base with marked areas of meningioma occurrence, A: olfactory groove, B: para- , suprasellar, C: petro-clival, D: sphenoid wing, E: foramen magnum.

5. Symptoms

In general, unspecific symptoms like headache might occur years before a correct diagnosis. Contrarily to tumours of the convexity, seizures are rarely seen in skull base meningiomas. Amongst skull base meningiomas seizures mostly happen in cases of sphenoid wing tumours.

5.1 Frontal skull base

Meningiomas developing at the frontal skull base, especially in the olfactory groove can be of grotesque size (Fig. 2) before diagnosed, due to the fact that hypo- or anosmia, may occur very slowly and thus might not impact the patients' life quality immediately. When spreading along the midline and reaching the tuberculum sellae other neurological symptoms may occur. Affection of the fronto-basal lobe can induce incontinence as well as psychotic disturbances, e.g. personality changes, psycho-motor disabilities and cognitive impairment. Visual disturbances occur due to compression of the optic nerve (reduction of vision, blindness) or affection of the chiasm (bitemporal hemianopsia). Furthermore, the compression of the pituitary stalk and/or the hypothalamus can induce endocrinological disturbances.

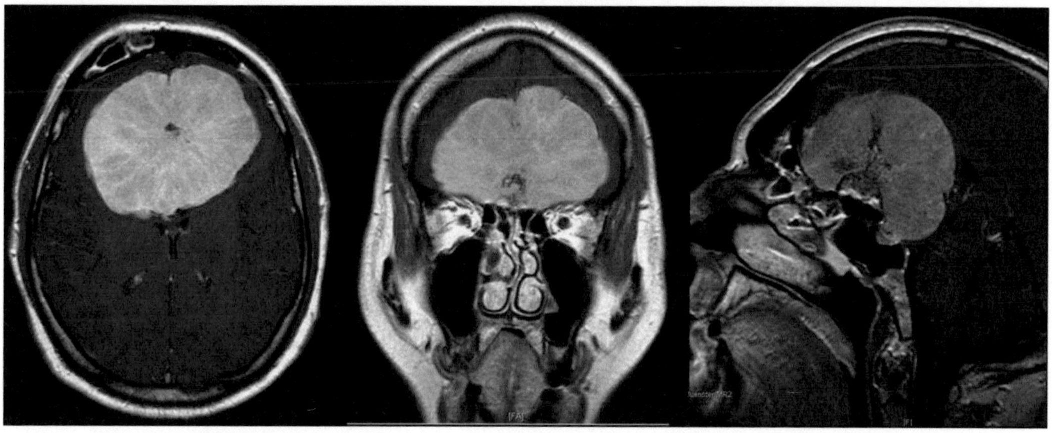

Fig. 2. T1-weighted triplanar magnetic resonance tomography after application of gadolinium, revealing a huge tuberculum sellae meningioma with homogenous contrast enhancement

5.2 Sphenoid ridge

Tumour growth along the sphenoid wing can cause a range of different neurological symptoms. When spreading into the middle skull groove, affecting the basal temporal lobe, seizures may be the first symptoms of the tumour. Furthermore, affection of the optic nerve can induce visual disturbance. Diplopia may occur due to compression of eye movement nerves (CN III, IV, VI), trigeminal nerve impairment may induce dysesthesia and/or loss of sensibility and ultimately even lead to a keratitis.

Especially bone invading sphenoid wing meningiomas might cause hyperostosis (Bikmaz et al. 2007).

5.3 Petro-clival

Tumour extension along the clivus may affect cranial nerves (CN V, VII-XI). According to the tumour mass and location (Fig. 3) occlusive hydrocephalus may occur as well as symptoms of brain stem compression (mono- or hemiparesis, paresthesia).

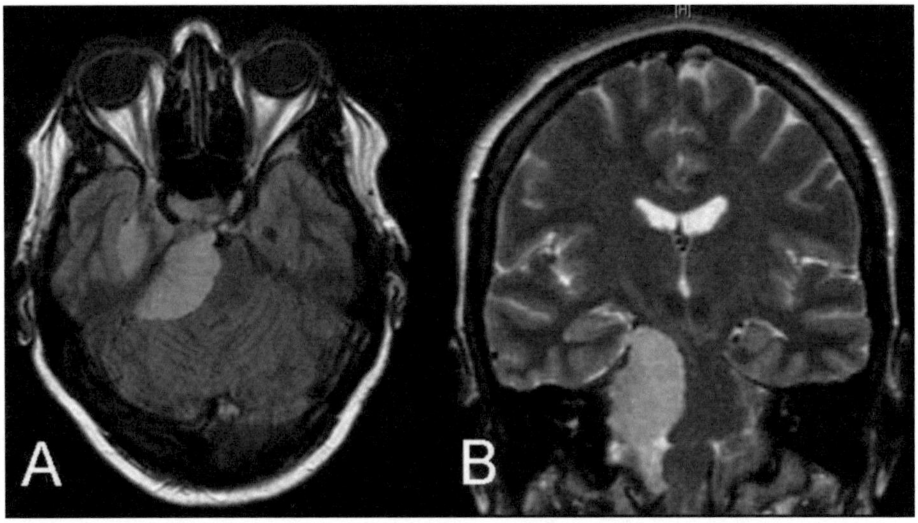

Fig. 3. Magnetic resonance tomography (A: T1 weighted, B: T2 weighted, both after application of gadolinium), showing a right sided petro-clival meningioma.

5.4 Foramen magnum

Meningiomas growing within the foramen magnum, ventral, lateral or dorsal, may affect especially the lower CN as well as brain stem functions. In addition to that occlusive hydrocephalus due to compression of the aqueduct may occur. Furthermore, meningioma within the posterior fossa, growing from the tentorium may compress and/or invade the cerebral sinus or arteries.

All tumours within the posterior fossa may irritate cerebellar functions, inducing ataxia, dysmetry, tremor and vertigo.

6. Pre-operative management

6.1 Neuro-imaging

In most patients with acute symptoms like seizures, a native computed tomography will be performed. In case of suspected intracranial or intracerebral mass and in absence of contraindications, a contrast-CT can be added. While classical indications as calcifications, surrounding edema and hyperostosis are revealed by native CT, tumour extension is well documented by a contrast-CT (Fig. 4). Performing an angio-CT may reveal the correlation between meningioma and vessels (Fischer et al. 2009). Assuming a sinus invasion more information can be gathered by angiography, especially in a venous phase.

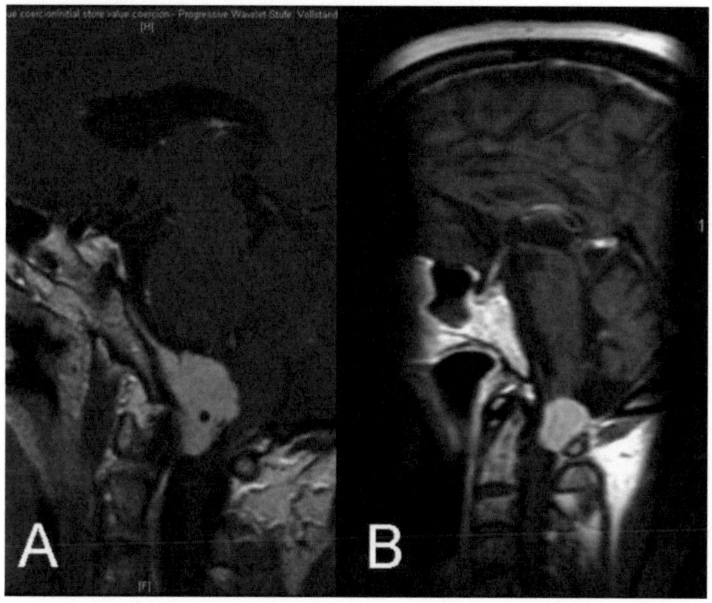

Fig. 4. Magnetic resonance tomography (coronar, T1-weighted, after application of gadolineum), showing **A**: a ventro-lateral and B: a dorso-lateral foramen magnum meningioma.

Magnetic resonance tomography including T1- and T2- weighted sequences, before and after contrast application, should be best practice in pre-operative meningioma diagnostic (Fig. 5).

In highly vascularized meningioma the demonstration of vascular architecture, e.g. by digital subtraction angiography, might be indicated to prevent vascular damage (Dowd et al. 2003). In special cases embolization of feeding arteries reduces the risk of disproportional intra-operative bleeding. Yet, there is no distinct data stating a definite duration between embolization and surgery, preventing re-opening of arteries as well as vascular genesis, which can sweep off the embolization effect (Dowd et al.2003).

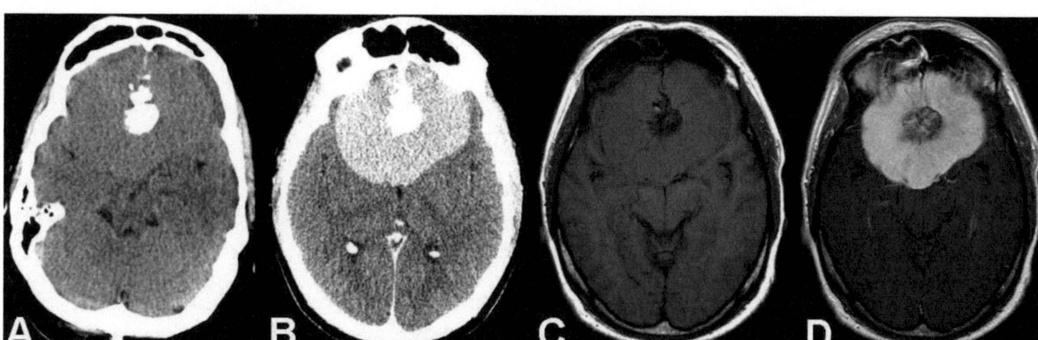

Fig. 5. Computed tomography (A: native and B: with contrast) and magnetic resonance imaging, T1 weighted (C before and D after gadolinium) revealing a huge tuberculum sellae meningeoma with central calcification and homogenous contrast enhancement (B, D).

6.1.1 Neuro-navigation

Technical innovations, such as neuro-navigation and intraoperative ultrasound led to more efficient planning of the surgical approach, due to smaller skin incision and bone resection. As ultrasound may show subcortical tumour localisation and vascularitiy and especially the course of larger vessels and tumour extension can be detected more easily. Other than in patients with sub-cortical tumours, in scull base meningiomas no brain shift occurs since the tumour is fixed at dural or osseous structures. In consequence, neuro-navigation may show the size of the residual tumour and the distance to vascular, neural and osseous structures.

For neuro-navigation 1 mm thick cranial CT-slices, scanned without gantry overturning, can be fusioned with MRI scans. This combination not only shows tumour mass, but also evidences vascular and neural structures as well as the extension within the osseous skull base.

Depending on tumour location and encasement of each cranial nerve, patients should be informed thoroughly about potential transient or persisting postoperative cranial nerve dysfunction. Appropriation of blood products (erythrocytes, thrombocytes) should be managed preoperatively.

6.2 Medication

- Steroids (e.g. dexamethasone 4mg q 8 hrs) are recommended to reduce peri-tumoural brain edema and edema-induced neurological symptoms
- Pre-operative application of anti-convulsive drugs is only indicated in patients with seizures and cannot be recommended prophylactically (Lieu&Howng 2000; Sughrue et al. 2011)
- Due to the possible distinct vascularization, impaired coagulation (e.g. pharmacologically by platelet aggregation inhibitors or coumarins) should not be present at time of surgery (Sughrue et al. 2011)

7. Approaches

In most cases of skull base meningiomas surgery is the first choice treatment. The success of surgical intervention depends substantially on the right approach to the tumour and thus substantially on the localization of the tumour.

Technical and medical advancement allow for the treatment of even deep or central seated meningiomas with low risk for peri-operative morbidity and mortality.

Since there are no strict recommendations on how to get access to the tumour, knowing the location of adjacent eloquent brain areas, run of cranial nerves, arteries and veins is essential to determine the most efficient and safe approach.

In this chapter we will describe some efficient approaches for treating skull base meningiomas of all kinds of localisations surgically. Anyways, best advice remains: "use the approaches you are familiar with".

In general, administration of hyperosmolaric fluids 30 min before skin incision, is recommended to all patients with skull base meningiomas unless there is no contraindication.

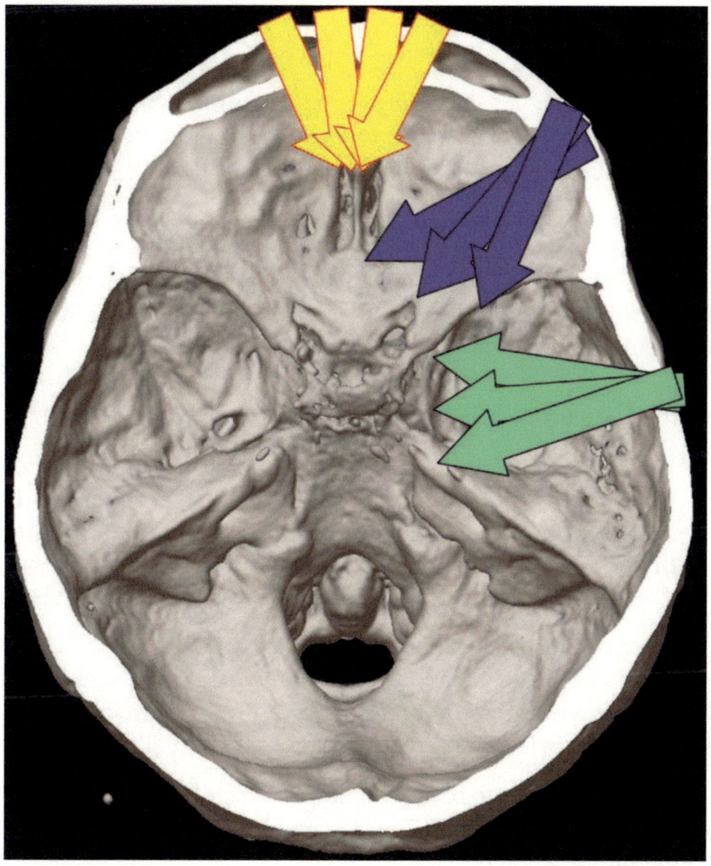

Fig. 6. Drawing of main approaches to meningiomas located in the olfactory groove, planum sphenoidale, para- and supra-sellar, sphenoid wing

7.1 Olfactory groove-, tuberculum sellae- meningiomas

In patients with olfactory groove meningiomas a fronto-basal craniotomy, mono- or bifrontal, and interhemispheric subfrontal approach is sufficient (Nakamura et al. 2006, 2008). For an interhemispheric approach occlusion of the superior sagittal sinus is sometimes necessary. In most cases this occlusion is without squeals if performed in the frontal third. A pre-operative CT-scan or digital subtraction angiography can reveal bridging veins, leading to the superior sagittal sinus, which should be preserved.

Dura opening should be semicircular with fronto-basal base.

7.2 Tuberculum sellae-, planum sphenoidale- meningiomas

Even though tuberculum sellae meningiomas are midline skull base tumours, the craniotomy for these tumours is placed supra-orbital reaching the tumour sub-frontally (Samii & Gerganov 2008). After dura opening, basal cisterns should be opened and CSF can be aspirated. Thus, by additional use of hyperosmolaric fluids and aspirating CSF the tumours can be reached with only slight retraction of the frontal lobe.

7.3 Sphenoid wing meningiomas

For small medial sphenoid wing meningiomas a supra-orbital craniotomy or a subfrontal approach are mostly used. Due to the extension of the tumour the supra-orbital craniotomy can be expanded to a orbito-zygomatic or a fronto-temporal craniotomy (Mahmoud et al. 2010; Seckin et al. 2008). Dura opening and CSF leakage should be performed like shown above.

Tuberculum sellae as well as sphenoid wing meningiomas sometimes invade the optic canal. In all cases of tumour extension into the optic canal, revealed by neuro-imaging pre-operatively, the nerve should be unroofed and tumour mass removed (Mahmoud et al. 2010). Otherwise swelling of residual tumour mass within the canal after closure of tumour vessels, especially veins, may deteriorate the visual faculty.

7.4 Petro-clival meningiomas

A multiplicity of approaches has been developed and is used today, depending on the extension of the tumour, the clinical status of the patient and especially the surgeon's experience. These approaches not only involve pterional and orbitozygomatic craniotomies but also sub-occipital approaches, sometimes in combination with a petrosal approach (Bambakidis et al. 2007; Kandenwein et al. 2009; Samii & Gerganov 2008; Seifert 2010).

In order to reach petroclival meningiomas, we recommend a sub-occipital craniotomy. Depending on tumour localization (ventral, lateral or dorsal) and size, these tumours often affect lower cranial nerves and/or the brain stem. To avoid cranial nerve and brain stem damage and get a better overview, the approach can be extended to a "far lateral approach".

For surgery of the posterior skull base, e.g. for suboccipital craniotomies, the patient is bedded in "parkbench-position" (Fig. 7). The endo-tracheal tube is combined with an electrode monitoring motor vagal nerve function.

In case of dorsal foramen magnum meningioma a partial laminectomy of the atlas is performed, if necessary with partial resection of the lamina of the axis.

In the pictures below craniotomy involves the foramen magnum as well as a partial resection of C1 in terms of partial laminectomy and mobilization of the vertebral artery (Fig. 8). Dura opening can be stretched across the complete cranio- and laminectomy. By preparing and opening of basal cisterns CSF can be withdrawn by suction.

A recently published comprehensive review on the outcome after surgery of petroclival meningeomas, stated no significant differences to the approach used (DiLuna & Bulsara 2010).

8. Intra-operative management

Skull base meningiomas often involve cranial nerves, brain arteries and might furthermore compresses the brain stem and/ or the spinal cord (DiLuna & Bulsara 2010). To avoid nerve and/or spinal cord injury, monitoring of nerve and spinal cord function is essential. In order to preserve motor cranial nerves electromyography should be recorded, furthermore visual, auditory, somato-sensory or motor evoked potentials should be monitored to avoid the nerve conduction (Topsakal et al. 2008). In all cases the efficiency of neuro-monitoring depends mainly on the kind of anaesthesia, therefore total intravenous anaesthesia should be used.

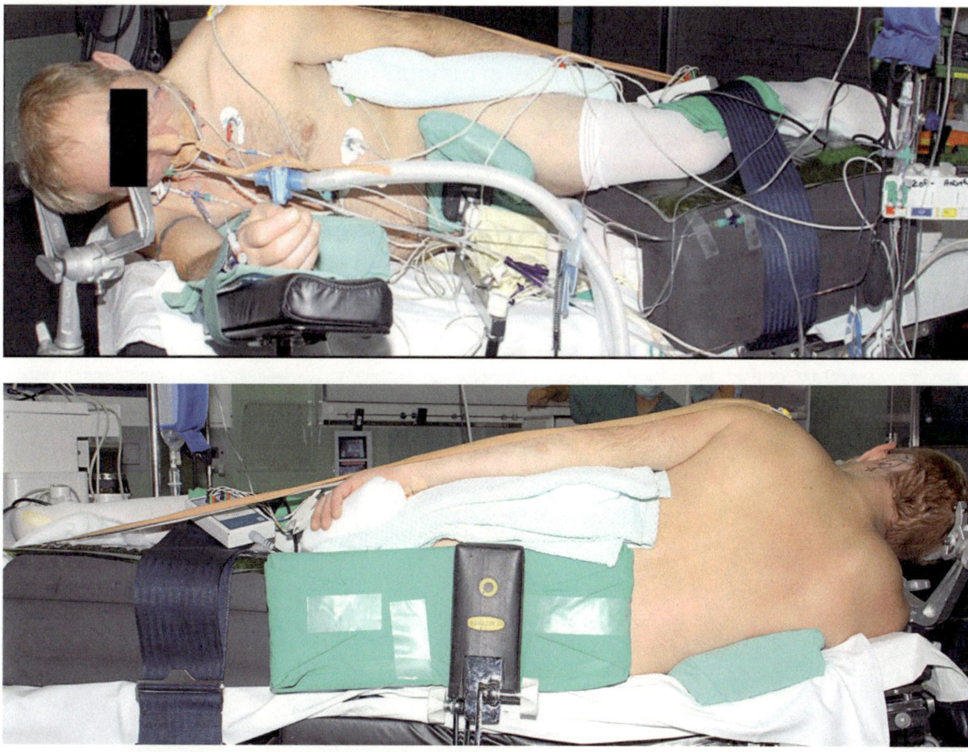

Fig. 7. For suboccipital approaches patients are bedded in park-bench position.

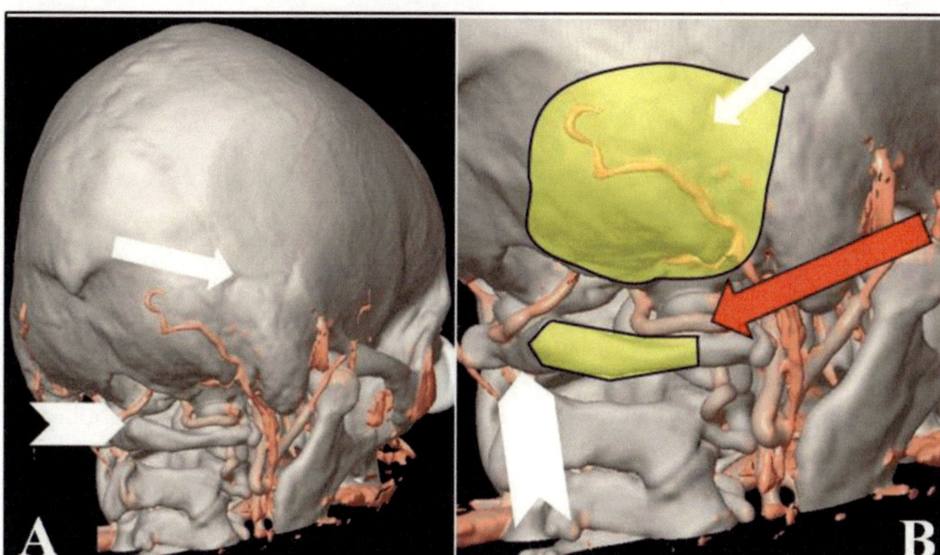

Fig. 8. Reconstruction of cranial computed tomography demonstrating the far lateral approach, **B** is an excerpt of **A**. Yellow areas highlight the extend of craniotomy and hemilaminectomy of the atlas (open arrow), after mobilization of the vertebral artery (red arrow). The keyhole for suboccipital craniotomy is placed on the asterion (closed white arrow).

8.1 Tumourresection

Since nervefibres may run within the capsule, in tumours affecting cranial nerves, these should be identified by neurostimulation to prevent neural deficit. Resection of the tumour then starts with opening of the tumour capsule and intracapsular debulking. To avoid damage of neural function due to traction and compression by manipulation, an ultrasound aspirator system is used. In many cases vascular supply of the tumour comes from arteries at the tumour basis and can not be cut off in the beginning of tumour resection. Furthermore, especially in petroclival meningiomas blood supplying arteries arising from different vascular territories have to be prepared carefully to prevent cerebellar or brain stem ischemia. Finally the capsule, after separation of nerves and vessels can be resected (Fig. 9).

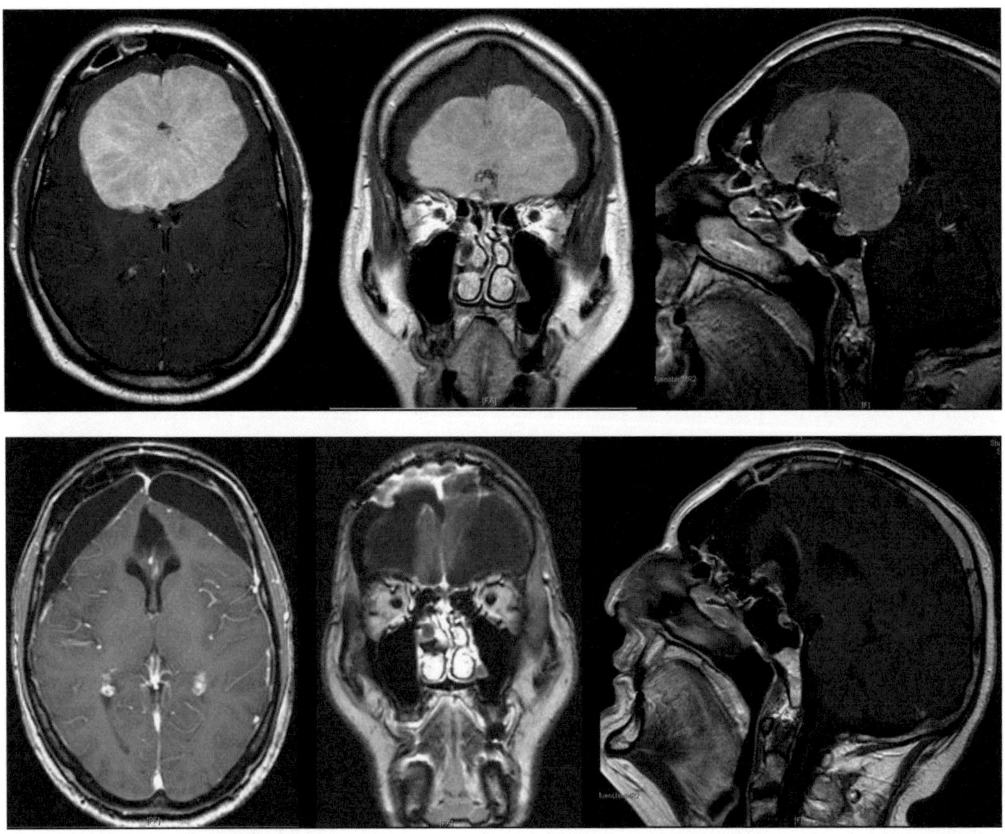

Fig. 9. Tri-planar, T1-weighted magnetic resonance imaging after gadolinium application, revealing nearly complete tumour removal (panel below) of the huge tuberculum sellae meningioma.

Whenever cranial nerves as well as vessels hinder tumour overview, new technical tools such as endoscopy may help to identify tumour residuals, especially in petro-clival meningiomas (Samii & Gerganov 2008). In selected patients, especially with frontal and tuberculum sellae meningiomas, endoscopic tumour removal with extended transnasal, transsphenoidal surgery, or with small craniotomy, can be successfully performed (Rachinger et al. 2010; Wang et al. 2010).

Similar to non skull base meningiomas, the grade of tumour resection is classified by the Simson grading system

Grade	Degree of removal
I	Macroscopically complete resection, excision of adjacent abnormal dura or bone
II	Macroscopically complete resection, coagulation of adjacent abnormal dura or bone
III	Macroscopically complete resection, no coagulation or excision of adjacent abnormal dura or bone
IV	Partitial removal
V	Decompression

Table 1. The Simpson grading system for removal of meningiomas (modified after Simpson 1957).

In different approaches, frontal, orbital, orbito-zytomatic as well as subocciptal, opening of frontal sinus or mastoid cells may occur. In such cases, mucosa has to be removed and the sinus as well as mastoid cells should be sealed with muscle or fat tissue and fixed with glue to avoid CSF leakage as well as inflammation.

Dural closure should be waterproof to prevent CSF leakage and re-operation. If dura was resected because of tumour invasion, dura plastic should be performed in an optimal way with autologous material such as galeal-periosteal flap.

9. Post-operative management

Post-operatively patients should be observed on an intense care unit where frequent neurological examination and optional mechanical ventilation is assured.

According to the extension of peri-tumoural edema steroid application should be continued for a few days, e.g. dexamethasone which is applicated 4mg q 8 hours the day of surgery and subsequently halved each following day.

Up to 25 % of meningioma patients develop seizures and antiepileptic drugs might be present in a large number of patients. Since intraoperative mechanical manipulation of the tumour surrounding brain tissue might even provoke further cortical epileptic activity, preoperatively onset antiepileptic drugs should be pursued for a few weeks postoperatively as well (Lieu & Howng 2000; Sughrue et al. 2011; van Breemen et al. 2007).

10. Adjuvant therapy

10.1 Radiation therapy

In patients with residual tumours as well as in patients with atypical or anaplastic meningiomas additional therapeutic options (radiotherapy, radiosurgery, e.g.) may help to control tumour growth and extension (Davidson et al. 2007; Minniti et al. 2009). With conventional fractionated radiotherapy, 50 - 55 Gy, admitted in 30 - 33 sessions, a local control rate is observed in about 80%, additionally tumour shrinking is seen in up to 25%

(Minniti et al. 2009). In cases of incomplete resected meningioma WHO grade I, adjuvant radiation therapy should be started if tumour re-growth is documented, whereas primary postoperative radiation therapy with 55 - 60 Gy should be initiated in patients with higher grade meningiomas, independent of resection grade.

The kind of used radiation technique depends on tumour size and localization and the distance between tumour and neural structures as for example the optic system. In meningioma greater than 4 ml and with a distance of more than 2 mm between tumour and neural structures fractionated stereotactic radiotherapy seems to be more efficient for tumour control than radiosurgery (Deinsberger & Tidstrand 2005).

Radiotherapy, e.g. radiosurgery, as first choice of treatment, may be indicated in patients not eligible for surgery due to co-morbidities, a tumour size less than 3 cm and/or tumour localization with high risk of intra- or post-operative vascular or neural damage (Davidson et al. 2007).

10.2 Chemotherapy

Medical therapy in patients with residual, inoperative or recurrent meningiomas has been subject of intense research. Due to the fact that meningiomas express progesterone receptors in up to 67% and somatostatin receptors in up to 100 %, chemotherapeutical studies focus on the development of receptor antagonists to stop tumor growth (Wen et al. 2010; Whittle et al. 2004). Yet, trials of various drugs have not been very successful (Norden et al. 2009, Schulz et al. 2011). Anyway, some data from ongoing and recently closed studies are still lacking, e.g. hydroxyurea (Norden et al. 2009; Newton et al. 2007). For additional therapeutic options such as receptor antagonists (vascular, angiogenesis, growth factor, hormones e.g.) the efficiency has to be revealed in clinical studies as well (Norden et al. 2009).

In all patients neuro-imaging controls should be performed periodically, at its best by MRI, the first one 3 month after surgery.

11. Outcome

In one study 5 year post-operative survival of meningioma patients was specified up to 91.3%. Anyway, recurrence rates and mortality are considerably affected by extent of surgical resection and histological grading. Analyses showed that WHO grade of skull base meningiomas is significantly lower as compared to their non skull base counterparts (Kane et al. 2011). Anyway, due to anatomical conditions resection of skull base meningioma still remains a surgical challenge and outcome is additionally affected by skills and experience of the treating surgeon as well as by exact tumour location and relation to adjacent anatomic structures. Subsequently, researching the literature reveals wide spreading postoperative morbidity and mortality rates.

In a current series of 73 sphenoid ridge meningiomas (Honig et al. 2010), rates of perioperative morbidity and mortality were 7% and 3%, respectively, with 11 patients (15%) developing tumour recurrence (mean follow-up 29.8 months). In another series of 117 foramen magnum meningiomas, perioperative mortality was 1.8%, recurrence rate among the 93 followed up patients was calculated for 1.1% (Wu et al. 2009). Concerning meningiomas of the ventro-medial skull base, analyses revealed gross total resection (simpson I and II) in approximately 90% with a perioperative mortality of 2.8% and recurrence rates 4.9% for both olfactory groove and tuberculum sellae meningiomas (Nakamura et al. 2006, 2008; Spektor et al. 2005). Additionally, table 2 gives an overview depicting morbidity and mortality following surgery for skull base meningiomas basing on a review of Chen et al. which mainly included outcome reports published from 2000 to the present (Chen et al. 2011) .

Location	Rate of total excision	Recurrence	Morbidity	Mortality
Anterior fossa	85–100%	0–4.9, mean follow-up of 2–5.28 years	0–31.3%	0–4.9%
Tuberculum sellae	76.4– 93%	1.4–4.2%, mean follow-up of 2.5–4.3 years	25–45%	0–8.7%
Medial sphenoid ridge	58–87%	0–9%, mean follow-up of 3.1–12.8 years	5.7–13%	0
Clinoidal	54.5–86.7%	3.8–15%, mean follow-up of 3.1–4.5 years	4–29%	0
Middle fossa, Cavernous sinus	0	5–5.7%, mean follow-up of 2.3–3.8 years	7.5–15%	0
Posterior fossa, Petroclival	0–48%	5–29%, mean follow-up of 3.9–8.5 years	20.3-47%	0–0.7%
Cerebellopontine angle	82–86.1%	3.9–7.5%, mean follow-up of 3.0–6.0 years	10.4–35.7%	0–5%
Foramen magnum	67–96%	0–5.5%, mean follow-up of 3.6– 6.1 years	5.9–27%	0–4.9%
Jugular foramen	50–100%	0–16.6%, mean follow-up of 2.5–6.5 years	30–61.5%	0–20%
Tentorial	77–91.3%	0–8.6%, mean follow-up of 4.5–5.9 years	9.7–55%	0–3.7%

Table 2. Outcome after surgical resection of skull base meningiomas of different locations (modified after Chen et al. 2011).

In order to estimate risk of meningioma surgery preoperatively, studies showed several predictors like patients' age, co-morbidity, preoperative neurological deficit, tumour size and location (Caroli et al. 2005; Joung & Lee 2008). Considering skull base lesions, Adachi et al. developed an ABC Surgical Risk Scale introducing a scoring system including previous radiation or tumour surgery, tumour attachment size, arterial involvement, brainstem contact, central cavity location and cranial nerve group involvement as predictors for a worse neurological outcome (table 2). Thus, score reaches from 0 to 12 points, which was subsequently graduated into low (0-4), moderate (5-7) and high (8-12 points) risk group compared to extend to surgical resection and patients´ outcome (Tabl. 3, Adachi et al. 2009). Although estimation of perioperative risk might still remain individual in most instances, this considerably depicts necessity of adequate preoperative imaging.

		Points		
		0	1	2
A	Attachment size	<2cm	2-4cm	>4cm
	Arterial involvement	None	Single	Multiple
B	Brainstem contact	CSF space visible	No CSF space visible	Perifokal edema
C	Central Cavity	Outside	Partitial involvement	Inside
	Cranial nerve group involvement	None	One	≥2

Table 3. The ABC Surgical Risk Scale for skull base meningioma CSF=Cerebrospinal fluid (modified after Adachi et al. 2009).

12. Future directions

Knowledge in underlying genetic alterations as well as in epigenetic pathologies is increasing and may help to identify genetic risk factors for tumour recurrence and malignancy (Bethke et al. 2008; Norden et al. 2009). Within the last years, new target therapy options such as hormone receptor antagonists and anti-angiogenetic drugs (e.g. bevacizumab) could be evaluated in meningioma therapy with partially results (Norden et al., Newton et al. 2007). Anyways, the role of such a specified target therapy remains unclear and needs to be determined in further investigations. Additionally, as compared to malignant gliomas, fluorescence-supported resection techniques might increase extend of tumour resection especially in cases of wide spreading dural and/ or bony infiltration with diffuse tumor borders. Depending on the varying fluorescence of meningiomas and its medicamentous persuasibility intraoperative, photodynamic therapy (PDT) might become a new therapeutic option especially for tumors of complex anatomical location like the skull base.

13. Summary and conclusion

Skull base meningiomas are no longer an unsolvable problem, due to technical advantages as well as new strategies in radio- and chemotherapy. Surgery, using all available technical tools, e.g. neuro-imaging, neuro-monitoring, has become effective and safe in aggressive tumour reduction and simultaneously in preservation of neural function. Moreover, even in residual, recurrent or malignant meningioma, adjuvant radiotherapy and prospective chemotherapy results in tumour control and sometimes in tumour shrinking.

Many patients with benign skull base tumours rather accept a residual tumour in combination with an adjuvant therapy and a normal nerve function, than a radical tumour resection with the consequence of an impaired nerve function.

14. References

Adachi, K.; Kawase, T.; Yoshida, K.; Yazaki, T. & Onozuka, S. (2009). ABC Surgical Risk Scale for skull base meningioma: a new scoring system for predicting the extent of tumor removal and neurological outcome. Clinical article. *J Neurosur,* 111, 5, pp. 1053-1061, ISSN 0022-3085.

Bambakidis, NC.; Kakarla, UK.; Kim, LJ.; Nakaji, P.; Porter, RW.; Daspit, CP. & Spetzler, RF. (2007). Evolution of surgical approaches in the treatment of petroclival meningiomas: a retrospective review. *Neurosurgery,*61, 5 Suppl 2, pp. 202-209, ISSN 0148-396X

Bethke L; Murray A; Webb E, et al. (2008). Comprehensive analysis of DNA repair gene variants and risk of meningioma. *J Natl Cancer Inst,* 100, pp. 270–276, ISSN 0027-8874

Bikmaz, K.; Mrak, R. & Al-Mefty, O. (2007). Management of bone-invasive, hyperostotic sphenoid wing meningioma. *J. Neurosurg,* 107, 5, pp. 905-912, ISSN 0022-3085.

Caroli, M.; Locatelli, M.; Prada, F.; Beretta, F.; Martinelli-Boneschi, F.; Campanella, R. & Arienta, C. (2005). Surgery for intracranial meningiomas in the elderly: a clinical-radiological grading system as a predictor of outcome. *J Neurosurg,* 102, 2, pp. 290-294, ISSN 0022-3085.

Chen, CM.; APH.; Lu-Ting Kuo, LT. & Tu, YT. (2011). Contemporary surgical outcome for skull base meningiomas. *Neurosurg Rev,* 34, 3, pp. 281-296, ISSN 0344-5607.

Chohan, MO.; Rehman, T.; Medina-Flores, R.; Clericuzio, C.; Heideman, R. & Marchand, E. (2011), 16 month-old female with intraventricular mass. *Brain Pathol,* 21, 3, pp. 349-50, ISSN 1015-6305.

Condra KS; Buatti JM; Mendenhall WM; Friedmann, WA.; Marcus, RB. & Rhoton, AL. (1997). Benign meningiomas: primary treatment selection affects survival. *Int J Radiat Oncol Biol Physiol,* 7, 39, pp. 427–436, ISSN 0360-3016.

Davidson, L.; Fishback, D.; Russin, JJ.; Weiss, MH.; Yu, C.; Pagnini, PG.; Zelman, V:, Apuzzo, ML. & Giannotta, SL. (2007). Postoperative Gamma Knife surgery for benign meningiomas of the cranial base. *Neurosurg Focus* 23, 4, E6, ISSN 1092-0684.

Deinsberger, R. & Tidstrand, J. (2005). Linac radiosurgery as a tool in neurosurgery. *Neurosurg Rev,* 28, 2, pp. 79-88, ISSN 0344-5607.

Diluna, ML. & Bulsara, KR. (2010). Surgery for petroclival meningiomas: a comprehensive review of outcomes in the skull base surgery era. *Skull Base,* 20, 5, pp. 337-342, ISSN 1531-5010.

Dowd, CF.; Halbach, VV. & Higashida RT. (2003). Meningiomas: the role of preoperative angiography and embolization. *Neurosurg Focus,* 15, 1, E10, ISSN 1092-0684.

Fischer, BR.; Palkovic, S.; Holling, M.; Niederstadt, T.; Jeibmann, A. & Wassmann, H. (2009). Coexistence of cerebral aneurysm and meningioma--pure accident? *Clin Neurol Neurosurg,* 111, 8, pp. 647-654, ISSN 0303-8467.

Honig, S.; Trantakis, C.; Frerich, B.; Sterker, I.; Kortmann, RD. & Meixensberger, J. (2010). Meningiomas involving the sphenoid wing outcome after microsurgical treatment-a clinical review of 73 cases. *Cen Eur Neurosurg,* 71, 4, pp. 189-98, ISSN 18684912.

Joung, H & Lee, BS. (2008). The novel "class" algorithmic scale for patient selection in meningioma surgery. In: Lee JH (ed) Meningiomas: diagnosis, treatment, and outcome. Springer, Berlin

Kandenwein, JA.; Richter, HP. & Antoniadis, G. (2009). Foramen magnum meningiomas--experience with the posterior suboccipital approach. *Br J Neurosurg,* 23, 1, pp. 33-39, ISSN 0268-8697.

Kane, AJ.; Sughrue, ME.; Rutkowski, MJ.; Shangari, G.; Fang, S.; McDermott, MW.; Berger, MS. & Parsa, AT. (2011). Anatomic location is a risk factor for atypical and malignant meningiomas. *Cancer,* 117, 6, pp.1272-1278, ISSN 1097-0142.

Lieu, AS. & Howng, SL. (2000). Intracranial meningiomas and epilepsy: incidence, prognosis and influencing factors. *Epilepsy Res* 38, 1, pp. 45-52, , ISSN 0920-1211.

Louis, DN.; Ohgaki, H.; Wiestler, OD.; Cavenee, WK.; Burger, PC.; Jouvet, A.; Scheithauer, BW. & Kleihues, P. (2007), The 2007 WHO classification of tumours of the central nervous system. *Acta Neuropathol,* 114, 5, pp. 97–109, ISSN 0001-6322.

Mahmoud, M.; Nader, R. & Al-Mefty O. (2010). Optic canal involvement in tuberculum sellae meningiomas: influence on approach, recurrence, and visual recovery. *Neurosurgery* 67, 3 Suppl, pp. 108-118, ISSN 0148-396X.

Mendenhall, WM.; Friedmann, WA.; Amdur, RJ. & Foote, KD. (2004). Management of benign skull base meningiomas: a review. *Skull Base,* 14, 1, pp. 53-60, ISSN: 1531-5010.

Michaud, DS.; Gallo, V.; Schlehofer, B.; Tjønneland, A.; Olsen, A.; Overvad, K.; Dahm, CC.; Kaaks, R.; Lukanova, A.; Boeing, H.; Schütze, M.; Trichopoulou, A.; Bamia, C.; Kyrozis, A.; Sacerdote, C.; Agnoli, C.; Palli, D.; Tumino, R.; Mattiello, A.; Buenode-Mesquita, HB.; Ros, MM.; Peeters, PHM.; van Gils,CH.; Lund, E.; Bakken, K.; Gram, IT.; Barricarte, A.; Navarro, C.; Dorronsoro, M.; Sánchez, MJ.; Rodríguez, L.; Duell, EJ.; Hallmans,G.; Melin, BS.; Manjer, J.; Borgquist, S.; Khaw, KT.; Wareham, N.; Allen, NE.; Tsilidis, KK.; Romieu, I.; Rinaldi, S.; Vineis, P. & Riboli, E. (2010). Reproductive factors and exogenous hormone use in relation to risk of glioma and meningioma in a large European cohort study. *Cancer Epidemiol Biomarkers Prev,* 19, 10, pp. 2562–2569, ISSN 1055-9965.

Minniti, G.; Amichetti, M. & Enrici, RM. (2009). Radiotherapy and radiosurgery for benign skull base meningiomas. *Radiat Oncol* 14, 4, 42, ISSN 1748-717X.

Nakamura, M.; Roser, F.; Struck, M.; Vorkapic, P. & Samii, M. (2006). Tuberculum sellae meningiomas: clinical outcome considering different surgical approaches. *Neurosurgery,* 59, 5, pp. 1019-1028, ISSN 0148-396X.

Nakamura, M.; Struck, M.; Roser, F.; Vorkapic, P. & Samii, M. (2008). Olfactory groove meningiomas: clinical outcome and recurrence rates after tumour removal through the frontolateral and bifrontal approach. *Neurosurgery,* 62, 6 Suppl 3, pp.1224-1232, ISSN 0148-396X.

Newton, HB. (2007). Hydroxyurea chemotherapy in the treatment of meningiomas. *Neurosurg Focus,* 23, 4, E11, ISSN 1092-0684.

Norden, AD. Drappatz, J. & Wen, PY. (2009). Advances in meningioma therapy. *Curr Neurol Neurosci Rep,* 9, 3, pp. 231-240, ISSN 1528-4042.

Rachinger, W.; Grau, S. & Tonn JC. (2010). Different microsurgical approaches to meningiomas of the anterior cranial base. *Acta Neurochir*, 152, 6, 931-9, ISSN 0001-6268.

Rockhill, J.; Mrugala, M. & Chamberlain, MC. (2007). Intracranial meningiomas: an overview of diagnosis and treatment. *Neurosurg Focus,* 23, 4, E1, ISSN 1092-0684.

Samii, M. & Gerganov, VM. (2008). Surgery of extra-axial tumors of the cerebral base. *Neurosurgery,* 62, 6 Suppl 3, pp. 1153-1166, ISSN 0148-396X.

Schulz, C.; Mathieu, R.; Kunz, U. & Mauer, UM. (2011). Treatment of unresectable skull base meningiomas with somatostatin analogs. *Neurosurg Focus,* 30, 5, E11, ISSN 1092-0684.

Seckin, H.; Avci, E.; Uluc, K.; Niemann, D. & Baskaya, MK.(2008). The work horse of skull base surgery: orbitozygomatic approach. Technique, modifications, and applications. *Neurosurg Focus,* 25, 4,E4, ISSN 1092-0684.

Seifert, V. (2010). Clinical management of petroclival meningiomas and the eternal quest for preservation of quality of life. *Acta Neurochir,* 152; 7, pp. 1099-1116, ISSN 0001-6268.

Simpson, D. (1957). The recurrence of intracranial meningiomas after surgical treatment. *J Neurol Neurosurg Psychiat,* 20, 1, pp. 22–39, ISSN 0022-3050.

Spektor, S.; Valarezo, J.; Fliss, DM.; Gil, Z.; Cohen, J.; Goldman, J. & Umansky, F. (2005). Olfactory groove meningiomas from neurosurgical and ear, nose, and throat perspectives: approaches, techniques, and outcomes. *Neurosurgery,* 57, 4 Suppl, pp. 268-280, ISSN 0148-396X.

Sughrue, ME.; Rutkowski, MJ.; Shangari, G.; Chang, HQ.; Parsa, AT.; Berger, MS. & McDermott, MW. (2011) Risk factors for the development of serious medical complications after resection of meningiomas. *J Neurosurg,* 114, 3, pp. 697-704, ISSN 0022-3085.

Topsakal, C.; Al-Mefty, O.; Bulsara, KR. & Williford, VS. (2008). Intraoperative monitoring of lower cranial nerves in skull base surgery: technical report and review of 123 monitored cases. *Neurosurg Rev,* 31, 1, pp. 45-53, ISSN 0344-5607.

Van Breemen, MS.; Wilms, EB. & Vecht, CJ. (2007). Epilepsy in patients with brain tumours: epidemiology, mechanisms, and management. *Lancet Neurol,* 6, 5, pp. 421-430, ISSN 1474-4422.

Wang, Q.; Lu, XJ.; Ji, WY.; Yan, ZC.; Ding, YS. & Zhang, J. (2010). Visual outcome after extended endoscopic endonasal transsphenoidal surgery for tuberculum sellae meningiomas. *World Neurosurg,* 73, 6, 694-700, ISSN 1878-8750.

Wen, PY.; Quant, E.; Drappatz, J.; Beroukhim, R. & Norden AD. (2010). Medical therapies for meningiomas. *J Neurooncol,* 99, 3, pp. 356-378, ISSN 0167-594X

Whittle, IR.; Smith, C.; Navoo, P. & Collie, D. (2004). Meningiomas. Lancet, 363, 9420, 1535-1543, ISSN 0140-6736.

Wiemels, J.; Wrensch, M. & Claus, EB. (2010). Epidemiology and etiology of meningioma. *J Neurooncol,* 99, 3, pp. 307-314, ISSN 0167-594X.

Wu, Z.; Hao, S.; Zhang, J.; Zhang, L.; Jia, G.; Tang, J.; Xiao, X.; Wang, L. & Wang, Z. (2009). Foramen magnum meningiomas: experiences in 114 patients at a single institute over 15 years. *Surg Neurol,* 72, , pp. 376-382 ISSN 1879-3339.

Yasargil, G. (1980). Meningiomas of the basal posterior cranial fossa. *Adv Tech Stand Neurosurg,* 7, pp. 1–115, ISSN 0095-4829.

6

Dural Reconstruction in Meningioma Surgery

Ciro Parlato[1], Roberto Granata[1], Aldo Moraci[1] and Marina Accardo[2]
[1]*Department of Neurosurgery,*
[2]*Department of Public Health Section of Pathology,*
Second University of Naples
Italy

1. Introduction

After many cranial and spinal neurosurgical removal of meningiomas, reconstruction of the dura mater is needed. The dura has to be meticulously closed following craniotomy (Protasoni et al., 2011), but primary dural closure with sutures alone can be difficult in a loss of native dural tissue (i.e., convexity meningiomas), to enlarge the dural compartment (i.e., inoperable intramedullary tumors) and when the closure is difficult and not sufficiently watertight because dura mater edges have shrunken and they cannot be sutured directly.

In this chapter we review different dural reconstruction techniques and we present our personal experience with TissuDura which is composed of colloidal collagen from equine Achilles' tendon and is inactivated with sodium hydroxide and chloridric acid. Unlike others dural substitutes who have different degrees of porosity, TissuDura has a lamellar structure that makes it waterproof, thus preventing the appearance of cerebrospinal fluid leak and tear. Previous reports have shown an absence of local and systemic toxicity and a low incidence of adherences and inflammation with TissuDura, making it a viable option for dural substitution. We present a series of patients who required dural graft implantation during various cranial and spinal neurosurgical procedures. Unlike previous reports, where a number of patients required sutures for fixation of the collagen matrix, our neurosurgical procedures were performed without the need for sutures, reducing surgery times, and allowing TissuDura to be applied to anatomically difficult locations. On the other hand we review different dural reconstruction techniques include watertight closure and nonwatertight closure of dural defects with and without dural grafts. Watertight closure of dural defects is required, as an inadequate closure of the dura mater at the end of neurosurgical procedures exposes the patient to cerebrospinal fluid leak, infections, hypertensive pneumocephalus, pseudomeningocele, cerebral herniation, and other complications that can lead to a longer period of hospitalization. Over the past decades, various types of material have been evaluated to determine the ideal dural replacement technique, including autografts, allografts, xenografts, and synthetic grafts. Neurosurgeons have used different types of graft to obtain an optimal duroplastic (Warren et al., 2000): egg membrane, rubber laminated leaf, gold foil and other materials. The first duraplasty described in literature was conducted in 1895 by Abbe. At the end of nineteenth century, Beach suggested the use of gold leaf to prevent the formation of meningocerebral adherences. However, many of these products have been associated with postoperative complications, some of which were serious, such as hemorrhages, development of corticomeningeal adhesions, inflammatory and foreign body reactions. Friction is the major complication of polytetrafluoroethylene duraplasty because of its strong surface tension and poor adaptability. Autologous duraplasties are accompanied by potential donor-site complications and are inappropriate for large defects. Acellular dermal grafts prepared from cadaver human skin do not suffer from these drawbacks; in addition, these matrices have been reported to promote the formation of new dural tissue by providing a scaffold for the growth of local cells while the matrix itself is fully reabsorbed over time (Islam et al., 2004). However, the use of human cadaver skin is associated with the development of atrophy or adhesion with the brain surface. Furthermore, relationships between iatrogenic Creutzfeldt–Jakob disease and implanted human cadaveric dura grafts have recently been reported. Similarly, implanted bovine xenografts carry a risk of transmission of bovine spongiform encephalopathy.

2. Dural substitutes

When primary closure is not possible, the use of dural grafts has been a common neurosurgical practice. This is the case especially in convexity meningioma surgery, where the removal of a large piece of dura along with the tumor to achieve a Simpson grade I or II resection results in a sizable defect that requires grafting. An ideal graft would show no inflammation in the host body and no neurotoxicity and adhesion to the underlying brain. At the same time it would be easily available and inexpensive, as well as durable, flexible, and easily prepared and shaped. Ideally, at the same time it would be rapidly resorbed, allowing the endogenous connective tissue to build up. Additionally, while providing adequate protection for the underlying brain, it should ensure watertight closure.

A common classification of dural substitutes includes: autografts (fascia lata, temporalis fascia), allografts (amniotic and placental membranes, pericardium, fascia, lyophilized dura), xenografts (bovine or porcine pericardium, peritoneum, dermis) and synthetic materials (polytetrafluoroethylene, polyester urethane). However, each materials pose drawbacks that limit their usage and require suturing to the endogenous dura to obtain a watertight closure.

2.1 Autografts

Autograft is a tissue that is taken from one part of a person's body and transplanted to a different part of the same person. There are several autografts, the most important of which are temporalis fascia, pericranium, autologous fat and fascia lata. Autografts do not transmit disease and do not give immuno-mediated responses in the host, but dimensions and qualities of tissues used for transplant are insufficient, especially when there is a considerable loss or retraction of dura mater. Furthermore, autograft requires an additional incision, resulting in an increase in surgical time with a consequent increase in anesthesic time, and a graft's hypoxia potentially causes an inflammatory response of underlying cortex (Islam et al., 2004).

Autologous fat is impervious to water, do not adhere to surrounding tissues and becomes revascularized (Black, 2010, as cited in Mayfield, 1980); it seems to be recommended for repair of dural tear or defects that are inaccesible or unsuitable for standard suture technique. However, autologous fat is not recommended in sovratentorial craniotomies (except in the evidence of a rhinorrhea after transsphenoidal approaches). Although rare, the most severe complications associated with autologous fat transplant are early fat necrosis and liquefaction (Hwang et al., 1996), fat dissemination in the subarachnoid space (McAllister et al., 1992) and subsequent lipoid meningitis (Ricaurte et al., 2000). Although causes of early fat necrosis are unknown, probably an initial transient ischemia determines early fat necrosis, followed by fat liquefaction. Moreover, liquefaction is more frequent and more serious in presence of a pathogen, in cerebrospinal fluid tear and leakage and after surgical wound's irradiation in postoperative time (Taha et al., 2011). Aseptic lipoid meningitis is the consequence of dissemination of liquefied fat into subarachnoid space, caused by the rupture of tumors or any event which weakens dura mater and creates a communication between epidural and subdural spaces. Differential diagnosis with other chemical meningitis is based on several clinical parameters that make lipoid meningitis easily distinguishable from other variants. In fact, lipoid meningitis occurs at least 1 week after surgery, does not respond to steroids and has a chronic and intermittent clinical course.

Pericranium (the external periosteum that covers the outer surface of the skull) is an autologous graft easy to harvest, does not require an additional skin incision and is more resistant to infection than synthetic grafts, but it is thin, fragile and difficult to handle. These difficulties could be overcome with the use of fibrin sealant; in fact, association of fibrin glue and pericranium seems to make it more easy to handle (Ito et al., 2011).

Despite having a sufficient thickness and being very tough, fascia lata (deep fascia of the thigh) is rarely used in neurosurgery because it is difficult to harvest and requires an additional skin incision, which determines an increased morbidity. On the other hand, temporalis fascia is a strong, fibrous graft used for duraplasty because it does not require an additional skin incision and has all the properties (thickness, strength, flexibility, easy availability) that makes it an optimal dural graft.

2.2 Allografts

Allograft is a transplant from one person to another, but not an identical twin. In past years, neurosurgeons have used several allogenic tissues for duraplasty (amniotic and placental membranes, pericardium, cadaveric lyophilized dura mater), many of which now rejected. Cadaveric lyophilized dura mater is a fragile tissue and creates adherences with sorrounding tissues and underlying brain; it can give immunomediated inflammatory reactions and trasmit Creutzfeldt - Jacob disease. In fact, it was hypothesized that prions could survive at any type of sterilization; however, it is important to remember that prions can be found in nervous system and have never been shown in dura mater. Moreover, re-operation have demonstrated atrophy of the allograft, even in well-performed surgery, and the transmission of Creutzfeldt - Jacob disease has created doubts about a possible viral transmission.

Dehydrated human pericardium, sterilized by γ-irradiation, is a valuable alternative when autologous material is not available: adherence to the cortex were not observed and dural patch was preserved and appeared as host dura (Caroli et al., 2004). Histologically they demonstrated a vascularization and fibroblastic infiltration of the dural substitute with good incorporation into the surrounding host dura). Moreover, its physical and mechanical properties make it an excellent choice.

Acellular dermal graft, derived from cadaveric human skin, has been used widely for various reconstructive surgery: it is tough, flexible, easy to suture, well tolerated and immunologically inert, does not create adherence with surrounding tissue and underlying brain, and form a watertight barrier that prevent cerebrospinal fluid leak. The internal structure of acellular dermal graft stimulates fibroblast invasion and rapid neovascularization without cell-mediated immune response (Chaplin et al., 1999): these characteristics justify the excellent rate of duralization of acellular dermal graft (Warren et al., 2000). Recently, some Authors have conducted an experimental study using 6 mongrel dogs (weight = 8-12 kg) and they have demonstrated that acellular dermal graft transplant has not been followed by infection, cerebrospinal fluid leak and adherence formation (Islam et al., 2004). Moreover, they histologically have found cellular infiltration of the graft: especially fibroblasts (mostly immature), neutrophils, rare monocytes and lymphocytes. They finally argue that acellular dermal graft may be a reasonable alternative to the available dural graft materials.

2.3 Xenografts

Bovine or porcine pericardium and other xenografts have been used as dural substitutes for many years. Equine Achilles' tendon, bovine or porcine pericardium are a surgical graft or tissue from one species to an unlike species. The prefix xeno- means foreign; it comes from the Greek word xenos, meaning stranger, guest, or host. There are two types of xenografts: 1) processed whole tissues; 2) highly engineered collagen matrix.

Bovine or porcine pericardium are examples of processed whole tissues. They are strong, pliable, easy to handle, economically advantageous, but require watertight suturing. Bovine pericardium is well tolerated, with a low incidence of postoperative complications (2%) (Hida, 2006, as cited in Laun, 1990); however, among the most common complication with this type of graft, there are the onset of foreign body reactions, aseptic meningitis and the transmission of Creutzfeldt - Jacob disease.

On the other hand, collagen matrix has several advantages: it serves as a scaffold and is completely replaced by patient's dura mater in few months (Narotam et al., 1995); moreover, it is an inert, elastic, easily handled adhesive material and does not cause inflammatory reaction or foreign body reaction. It is formed by type I collagen, a very insoluble and only weakly immunogenic material (Narotam, 2009, as cited in Ellingsworth, 1986); in fact, collagen immunogenicity is poor due to absence or scarcity of aromatic aminoacids (Reddy et al., 2002). Requiring no suture and using it as an onlay graft, collagen matrix reduces surgery time and the risk of foreign body giant cell reaction, a frequent complication when neurosurgeon have to suture dura mater (Narotam, 2009, as cited in Macfarlane, 1979). If the overlap between the graft and the dura is appropriate (minimum overlap required = 1 cm), collagen matrix can be used as an onlay graft without an additional fixation; otherwise neurosurgeon needs to use one or multiple additional fixation (for example, fibrin sealant). However, it seems that simultaneous multiple fixation are associated with a higher rate of infection and cerebrospinal fluid leaks (Stendel et al., 2008).

In summary, sutureless dural repair using collagen matrix has several advantages: reducing surgery time, facilitating application of small patches in surgical difficult location, overcoming difficulties related to presence of fragile or ossified dura mater. This advantages are fundamental in transsphenoidal approach for the narrowness of operative field: a duraplasty is necessary only when neurosurgeons demonstrate a cerebrospinal fluid tear or leak and when there is a communication between sovrasellar arachnoid cistern and sellar cavity (Biroli et al., 2008); in these cases surgeon can only use collagen matrix or associate it with a fibrin sealant. Recently, some Authors have demonstrated a lower operating time with the use of collagen matrix as compared with suturable acellular human dermal grafts (Danish et al., 2006).

2.4 Synthetic grafts

Synthetic graft are also widely used in Neurosurgery. In past years several materials have been introduced in surgical practice (polytetrafluoroethylene, polyester urethane). However, these materials present a lot of drawbacks that placed them in the background. Despite their theoretical uniform thickness and no risk of infection transmission, polytetrafluoroethylene and the other synthetic grafts have often a rigid structure, resulting difficult to handle, are often not able to be replaced by dura mater and are burdened by numerous inflammatory and foreign body reactions. These reactions can create an inflammation of surrounding tissues and underlying brain, an excessive fibrin production with graft encapsulation, cerebrospinal fluid bleeding, meningitis, graft rejection, scarring, infections, delayed bleeding, for which a reoperation is often required. Moreover, in watertight closure holes created by suturing graft to dura mater could cause a cerebrospinal fluid leakage. The strength of synthetic absorbable grafts is only guaranteed for the first 2 weeks: these materials are often brittle and they tends to give cerebrospinal fluid leaks, without preserving the guest from serious inflammatory reactions (Yamada et al., 1997). Other drawbacks of polytetrafluoroethylene are represented by its strong surface tension and its lack of adaptability, frequent appearance of friction injury with underlying brain and meninges, which may cause bleeding and inflammation (Islam, 2004, as cited in Yamagata, 1993). On the other hand, some Authors have evaluated advantages and drawbacks of a new synthetic dural graft, designed for use both in traditional watertight dural closure and as a dural underlay graft in non-watertight fashion (Chappell et al., 2009). This dural substitute has two different surfaces: the first one, placed in contact with the brain, is a porous structure (pores diameter < 1 μm, so that cellular migration and penetration are prevented); the second one has a porous structure too, but it has larger pores (diameter ~ 22 μm), resulting in a rapid cellular infiltration and migration. They finally argue that this synthetic graft may be used as an underlay graft to obtain a non-watertight closure. On the other hand, if used over large voids, watertight closure is also viable.

Moreover, a new transparent artificial dura mater derived from silk fibroin was recently evaluated in craniotomized rats (Kim et al., 2011). This synthetic graft seems to have an excellent biocompatibility, good water vapor and oxygen permeability, blood compatibility, and promotes collagen formation and proliferation of human fibroblast in vitro. The high tensile strength of this material allowed them to suture it easily to the rats' dura mater without demonstrated cerebrospinal fluid tear of leak. Although the Authors cannot establish long term effects of silk fibroin, they argues that its optimal biocompatibility and its ability to inhibit inflammatory reaction make it safe and potentially useful for future neurosurgery.

3. Surgical sealant

Surgical sealants (also called surgical glues or adhesives) are used after a surgery or traumatic injury to bind together external or internal tissue. Surgical glues can be used in conjunction with or as an alternative to sutures and staples; they use a chemical bond to hold tissue together for healing or serve as a barrier to stop the flow of bodily fluids. The four main types of surgical glues are fibrin sealants, cyanoacrylates, glutaraldehyde glues and hydrogels. Cyanoacrylates (stronger than fibrin sealants and sutures, waterproof, flexible) and glutaraldehyde glues (a pungent colorless and potentially neurotoxic oily liquid) are not used in neurosurgery.

3.1 Fibrin sealant

Fibrin sealants are a type of surgical adhesive derived from both human and animal (bovine) blood products. One of these glues is a two component fibrin sealant that consists of human fibrinogen and human thrombin. When combined, thrombin converts fibrinogen to fibrin forming a clot. The mechanism of action of this fibrin glue is expressed by a permanent and rapid adhesion between human tissues and graft, supporting or replacing conventional sutures; moreover, it stimulates haemostasis and dural replacement. These sealants are not neurotoxic: in fact subdural administration in the rabbit was not associated with any adverse reaction (Epstein, 2010). Because adverse reactions are reported voluntarily and the population is of uncertain size, it is not always possible to reliably estimate the frequency of these reactions. Adverse effects are represented by allergic reaction, which may include angioedema, bradycardia, bronchospasm, dyspnea, agitation, tachycardia, headache, hypotension, generalized urticaria, vomiting, but it occur rarely in patients treated with fibrin glue/haemostatic drugs. In isolated cases, these reactions have progressed to severe anaphylaxis. Accidental intravascular administration may cause anaphylactic reaction, thromboembolic complications and disseminated intravascular coagulation. Hypersensitivities to fibrin glues and bovine protein are the only contraindications.

3.2 Hydrogels

Hydrogels are FDA-approved synthetic polyethylene glycol polymers, stronger than fibrin sealants. They are synthetic absorbable sealants (that have to be added to sutured dural repair to obtain a watertight closure), work in the presence of fluid, conform to irregular surface, demonstrate strong adherence and compliance to tissues without interfering with underlying tissue visibility and are reabsorbed in 4-8 weeks without leaving residue. They are also photoactivated, meaning that the sealant sets with exposure to light, which can be a drawback in situations where a patient is hemorrhaging. Hydrogels manufacturer suggests to not apply this sealant to confined bony structures where nerves are present since neural compression may result due to hydrogel swelling (hydrogel may swell up to 50% of its size in any dimension). Other Authors argue the safety and efficacy of a polyethylene glycol hydrogel sealant in patients undergoing elective cranial surgery with documented cerebrospinal fluid leakage after sutured dural repair, when it was used as an adjunct to sutures (Cosgrove et al., 2007). Contraindications include allergy, renal or hepatic dysfunction, head trauma, infection, hydrocephalus, cranial procedure that entails a dural incision involving penetration of the air sinus or mastoid air cells and in a ventricular or lumbar drain. Moreover, hydrogel should not be used if an active infection is present at the surgical site, in patients with a compromised immune system or autoimmune disease and in combination with other sealants or haemostatic agents. Potential risks and adverse events that could occur from the use of hydrogels include, but are not limited to, wound infection, immediate, delayed and/or persistent cerebrospinal fluid leak, renal compromise, inflammatory reaction, neurological compromise, allergic reaction and/or delayed healing. A type of hydrogel was evaluated in 111 investigational patients in a pivotal clinical study, published in its own package leaflet. Adverse events (cerebral edema, cerebrospinal fluid leak, deep surgical site infection, headache, hydrocephalus, aseptic and bacterial meningitis, cognitive deficits, cranial nerve deficits, motor deficits, neuropsychiatric disorders, speech difficulty, visual disturbance) occur at a rate of 1% or higher in examined patients. Adverse event rates are based on the number of patients having at least one occurrence of a particular adverse event divided by the total number of patients treated. There were two patient deaths (out-of-hospital). In both cases, the deaths were attributed to the patients' prior condition. Recently, Epstein has reviewed literature and has demonstrated in two patients that the use of hydrogel was associated with quadriplegia and a cauda equina syndrome (Epstein, 2010).

4. Watertight closure

Duraplasty, like many surgical techniques and applications, is largely based on the personal experiences of individual surgeons, shaped by training passed down from mentors, and repeated generation after generation. The traditional teaching in neurosurgery has been that the dural reconstruction has to be watertight. This is fundamental (but sometimes very difficult to achieve) in meningioma surgery, especially when an extensive resection of a large convexity meningioma, a skull base meningioma or a posterior fossa meningioma with its dural tail is needed. A fundamental element of the watertight dural reconstruction is the use of suturing. Some Authors developed an in vitro model, testing different suturing techniques in providing watertight closure of the dura mater (Megyesi et al., 2004). They compared the efficacy of the interrupted simple, running simple, running locked, and interrupted vertical mattress sutures on primary closure of linear incisions and closure of dural defects using rectangular grafts. The results showed superiority of interrupted simple suture on primary closure of linear incisions over other techniques. In literature, the emphasis on watertight closure has been strong to the point that special techniques have been developed and proposed to reach difficult areas in order to achieve optimal dural reconstruction. However, one potential risk of using primary suture closure would be to create pinholes from the suture needle. In an attempt to achieve watertight closure, holes created on either side of the dura mater or the dural substitute may commonly lead to cerebrospinal fluid leakage. In addition, while implanting synthetic graft materials, dural tearing may be caused by the sutures themselves because of the elastic properties of these grafts which exert traction on the sutures. It is probably because of these factors that studies have shown up to sevenfold more favorable rates of effective dural closure when suture repair is augmented by tissue adhesives. To really understand limits created by the need to suture the dura mater, we make the example of duraplasty to repair a spinal cerebrospinal fluid tear or leak. A dorsal dural tear or leak can be repaired by applying direct sutures. However, lateral spinal dural tear create a technically difficult problem for placement of sutures because of its inaccessibility. The same problem is present in ventral dural tear or leak: suturing in this area may be a real challenge. However, surgeons can apply a large fat layer on the ventral surface of dural sac, suturing this autologous graft to the outer layer of the dura mater to create a reinforcement of spinal dural suture lines (Black, 2000).

5. Non-watertight dural reconstruction with collagen matrix

Recently, there has been an interest in processing tissues with high connective tissue components such as pericardium and dermis to yield an acellular, antigen-free scaffold for growing endogenous tissue. Other Authors use collagen matrix (DuraGen, Integra Neurosciences, Plainsboro, NJ) for dural reconstruction in the majority of meningiomas where dural enlargement or watertight closure are required. This material is made up of type I collagen and is processed from bovine Achilles' tendon. The collagen matrix provides a low-pressure absorptive surface to diffuse cerebrospinal fluid and attaches to the dural surface via surface tension. It also helps clot formation by the platelets depositing themselves on the collagen, which then disintegrate and release clotting factors, ultimately facilitating fibrin formation. This fibrin has an important role in holding the graft in place until fibroblasts, associated with blood vessels, proliferate into the graft. This fibroblast infiltration starts by day 3–4 and becomes established in 10–14 days. The fibroblasts use the pores on the matrix to lay down endogenous collagen. By 6–8 weeks, the collagen matrix is resorbed and is integrated to the endogenous dura. The non-watertight reconstruction of the dura using the collagen matrix simply consists of the onlay application of the material over the dura. It is easily shaped and has the main advantage of not requiring any suturing. The collagen matrix is incorporated in the endogenous tissue in a relatively short period of time and in 24 weeks becomes barely distinguishable from the endogenous dura, unlike the allogenic cadaveric dura, which shows inadequate fusion with the endogenous dura and in addition becomes encapsulated in a connective tissue layer. This encapsulation has also been described for synthetic materials, which appears not to be an ideal situation with regard to the sealing quality of the material. It has also been shown that the compact structure of the xenogenic materials may limit the fibroblast migration to the edges or to the suture holes. In addition, the collagen, in the form of sponge, can absorb fluid without increasing its volume, and can act as a moistening agent for the brain, allowing penetration of cerebrospinal fluid into the graft. It also forms an effective separation layer and minimizes adhesions between the brain and the overlying tissue. These Authors concluded that non-watertight reconstruction of the dura in meningioma surgery prevented postoperative cerebrospinal fluid leak in 99.6% of patients (Lee, 2008). Graft-related complication was seen in only 2 patients (0.8%). These figures compare favorably to the majority of the reported series in which various techniques of watertight closure is described and the indispensability of watertightness in dural closure is emphasized. In addition to the extremely low rate of graft-related complications and cerebrospinal fluid leak, this technique makes significantly shorter the operative procedure, thereby possibly decreasing the risk of anesthesia-related complications as well, which would be of particular concern in patients with medical comorbidities. It would even help reducing the medical costs related to shortened operating room usage.

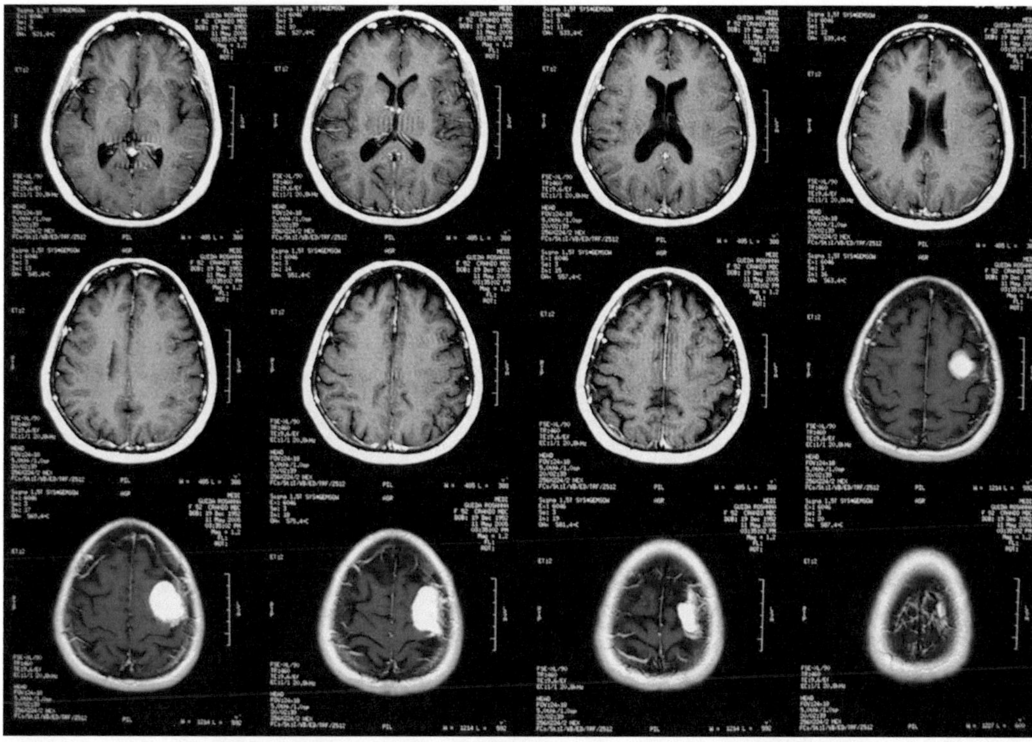

Fig. 1. Preoperative MR with gadolinium of left frontoparietal meningioma.

In our series, we analyzed dural reconstruction in 50 patients affected by meningiomas: 31 in the frontoparietal paramedian region and 19 in the parieto-occipital paramedian region. All cases of dural reconstruction were performed at our department of neurosurgery of the Second University of Naples between 2005 and 2009. TissuDura was rehydrated in physiological saline to obtain a transparent film that could be cut into the desired shape. Patches of the collagen matrix were cut with scissors to the appropriate size for the dural defects with an overlap of 1 cm. The patch was then placed over the dural defect, overlapping at the margins. The patch was fixed using fibrin glue. To avoid postoperative fibrosis, minimal amounts of fibrin glue were used in the repair of the dural defects. Surgical sutures were not used during dural reconstruction. No patient required removal of the graft, and the overlay technique with the use of fibrin glue was simple and fast. The time needed for the neurosurgical procedures was reduced. TissuDura facilitated the application of small patches in anatomically difficult locations. At follow-up, we did not observe any signs of graft rejection or cerebrospinal fluid leaks in any of our patients, and no other complications occurred. We observed the reorganization of dura and normal cerebrospinal fluid circulation. In the two cases of recurrent atypical meningioma, reoperation of the dural reconstruction was performed after 1 year. We observed no adherences between the brain and neodura. Neodura formation allowing fibroblast ingrowth and collagen formation was observed. In these cases, histopathological and ultra structural findings from the previously implanted TissuDura showed fibroblasts and new normal dural tissue. The collagen matrix was fully degraded and replaced by natural collagen. TissuDura was not recognized as a foreign material and no tissue reactions were observed. We used TissuDura in a wide range of spinal and cranial neurological procedures. Usually, dural reconstruction during spinal surgery must be meticulously sutured to avoid cerebrospinal fluid leaks because of the increased hydrostatic pressure in the supine or upright position; nevertheless, we performed the reconstructions without sutures and at follow-up we did not observe any cerebrospinal fluid leakages.

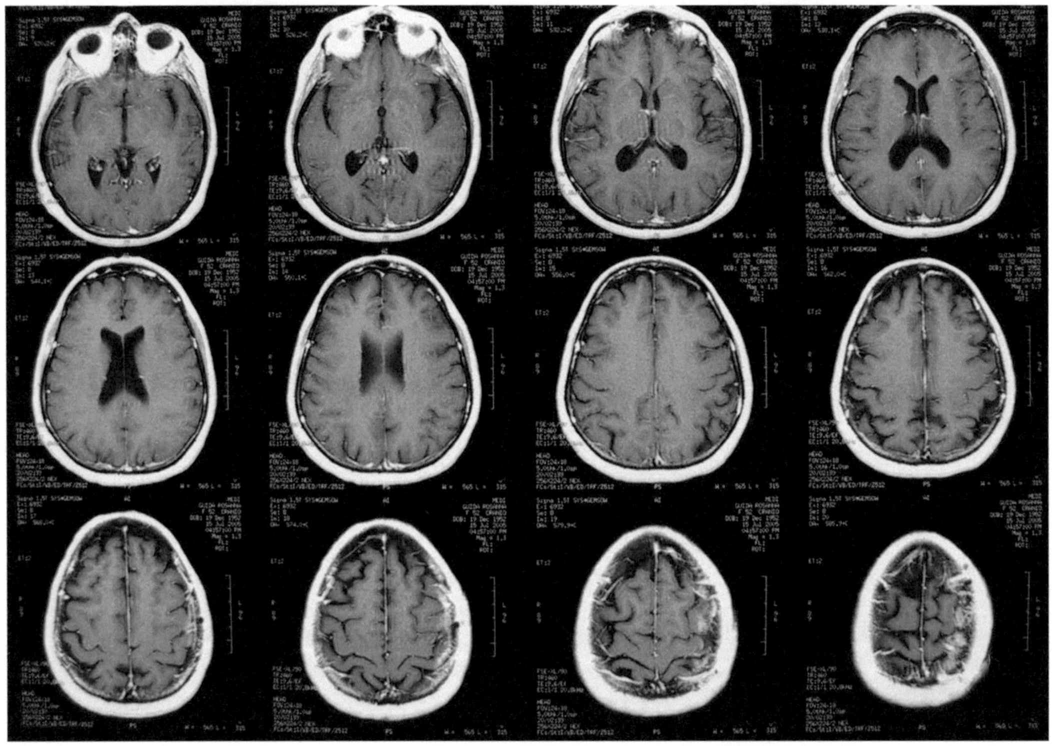

Fig. 2. Dural reconstruction by TissuDura and fibrin glue. Postoperative MR with gadolinium of complete removal of left frontoparietal meningioma.

The use of autologous fat transplants is recommended as a rapid, effective means for repair of dural tears or defects that are inaccessible or unsuitable for standard suture technique. TissuDura may be a viable alternative to these techniques. Some Authors developed a dural substitution technique using bio absorbable fabric and fibrin glue (Hida et al., 2006). In 160 patients who underwent dura repair using this polyglycolic acid–fibrin sheet method, ten (6.3%) experienced subcutaneous cerebrospinal fluid leakage. The Authors concluded that this technique represents a novel alternative to artificial dural substitutes that were available at that time. Recently, other Authors showed that collagen matrix is suitable for use in the posterior fossa where it can be applied as an onlay graft, without the inconvenience and time-consuming process of suturing (Narotam et al., 2007). This represents a more developed collagen-based dural graft compared with a collagen sponge; it was associated with a good safety profile, as well as being effective, easy to use, and time efficient. However, meticulous layered wound closure, the detection and effective control of hydrocephalus, and the use of closed suction wound drainage were required to minimize potential complications related to the use of collagen matrix duraplasty. In our patients, the overlay technique for dural reconstructions using TissuDura was easy and fast and allowed good results in dural repair during meningiomas surgery without the use of closed suction. To avoid postoperative fibrosis, we used a minimal amount of fibrin glue in the repair of the dural defects. Studies of intracranial implantation in adult sheep showed that implantation of collagen biomatrix did not result in inflammation, cerebrospinal fluid leaks, or impaired wound healing (Knopp et al., 2005). Microscopic assessment of graft incorporation 2 weeks postoperatively showed loosening of the homogeneous structure of the collagen graft with invasion of lymphocytic and monocytic components. After a period of 4 weeks, lymphocytic and monocytic exudates were present and polymorphonuclear giant cells were common with numerous fibroblasts. Eight weeks postoperatively, inflammatory infiltrates had regressed further. After 24 weeks, there was a further regression of inflammatory infiltrates and continuity between the highly collagenous endogenous dura and the newly formed collagen fibers of neodura. In another case report, histological examination of a tissue sample taken 40 days after implantation of a collagen matrix revealed that the graft had been replaced by significant ingrowth of the native dura (Gazzeri et al., 2009). Similarly, in our two patients with recurrent meningiomas who required re-operation, long-term follow-up using histopathological and ultra structural techniques demonstrated re-absorption of the TissuDura and regeneration of dura mater. The first report with documented histopathological and ultra structural imaging showing dura regeneration after TissuDura graft insertion was presented (Parlato et al., 2011). Our ultrastructural observations showed an absence of inflammatory infiltration and migration of fibroblasts, resulting in the neodura regeneration. The collagen matrix was fully degraded and replaced by native collagen neodura after 12 months.

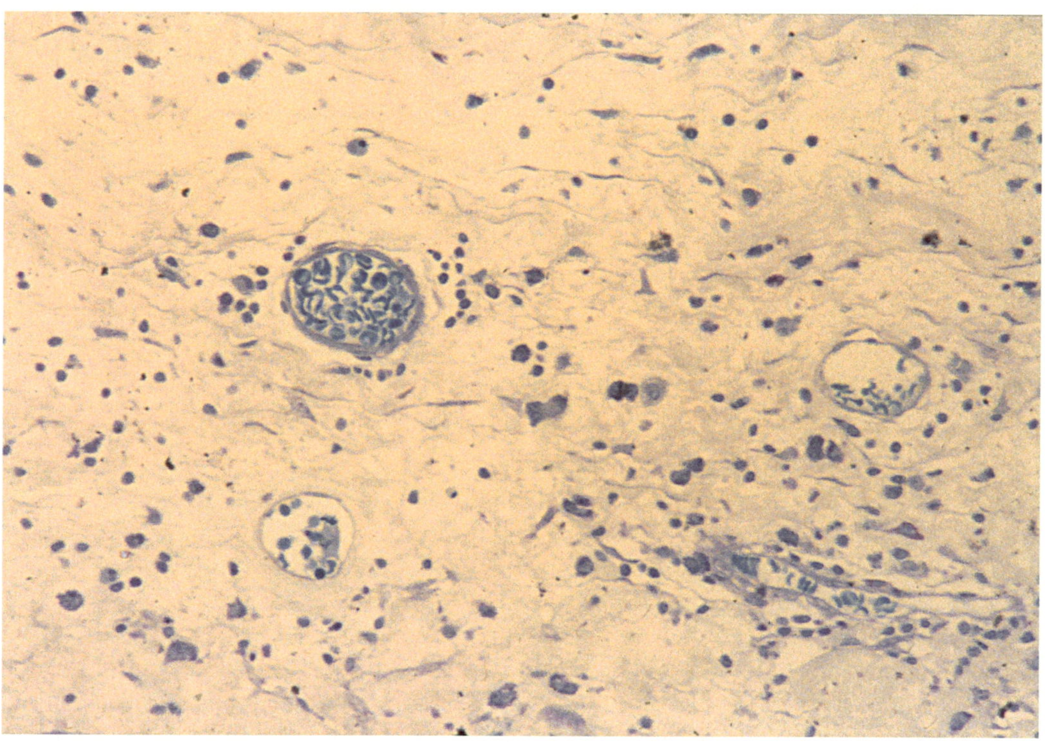

Fig. 3. Neurohistopathological photomicrographs of neodura.

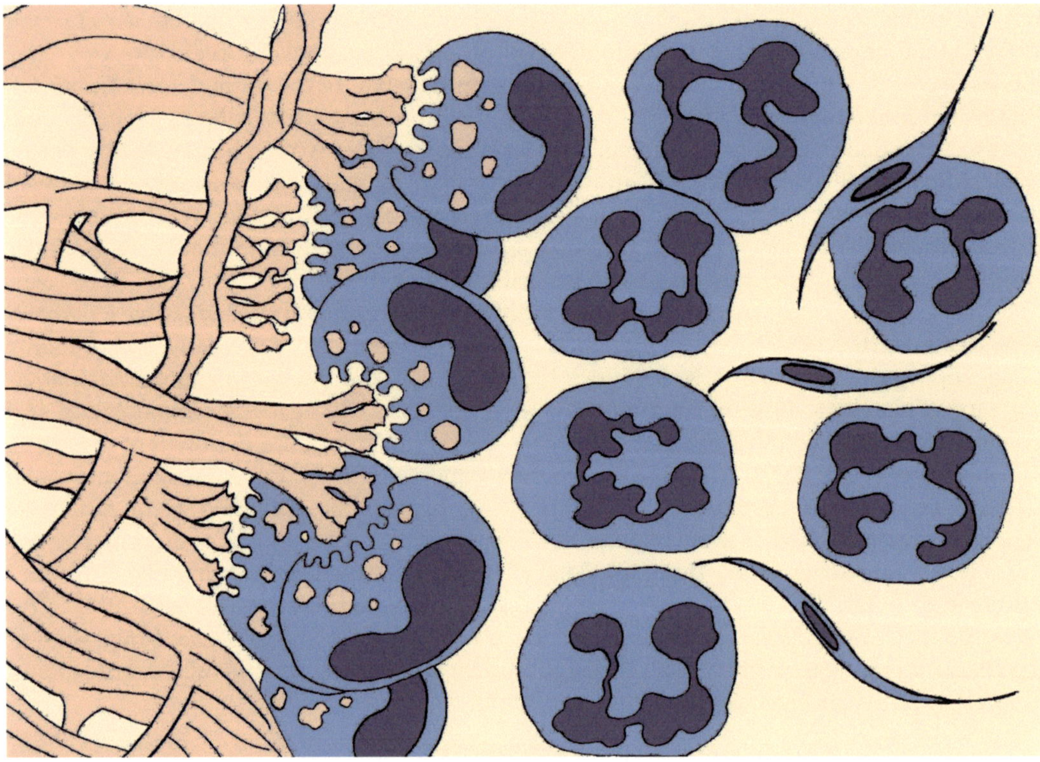

Fig. 4. Illustration of collagen matrix and its interaction with macrophages and neodura.

TissuDura demonstrated all aspects of the ideal dura substitute: elasticity, nonreactivity, good adaptability, and easy and speed of application. Dural reconstructions were performed without surgical sutures, and no incidences of local toxicity or complications such as cerebrospinal fluid leaks, adherences, or inflammation were observed. Moreover, the overlay technique with the use of fibrin glue was simple and quick to perform. Histopathological and ultra structural images demonstrated dura regeneration after TissuDura graft insertion in patients with recurrent meningioma after 12 months follow-up.

6. Duraplasty after transsphenoidal approach

The transsphenoidal approach is a minimally invasive surgical technique for the removal of several tumors; in this chapter we examined dural reconstruction after surgery of tuberculum sellae, olfactory groove and clival meningiomas. The evolution of the technique has coincided with progress in biotechnology. In the early twentieth century, Hirsh and Cushing have designed and demonstrated benefits of transsphenoidal surgery compared to the classical transcranial approach. Subsequently, Dott, a Cushing's assistant, have ideated several instruments to improve the use of this technique. In 1967, Hardy have used operating microscope for the first time. This progress has been joined by surgeons over the years, making transsphenoidal surgery safer and less invasive. In particular, tuberculum sellae meningiomas are suprasellar meningiomas, frequently arise from the tuberculum sellae, chiasmatic sulcus, Planum sphenoidale, and diaphragma sellae and comprise 5% to

10% of all intracranial meningiomas (Bassiouni et al., 2006). There are several surgical advantages of the endoscopic endonasal transsphenoidal approach for the improvement of visual outcome and the surgical treatment of tuberculum sellae meningiomas (Wang et al., 2010). First, the most important advantage is the avoidance of manipulation of an ischemic, compressed optic system. Second, the extended endoscopic endonasal transsphenoidal approach provides the potential for early and direct visualization of subchiasmatic perforators. Third, complete mobilization and decompression of the optic nerve contribute to its protection. Fourth, this approach obviates brain retraction, provides better cosmetic results in addition to increased patient comfort, and permits working under direct visual control to realize a Simpson grade I removal (Jallo et al., 2002). Recently, advantages and drawbacks of Extended Transtuberculum Transplanum Approach (ETTA) are examined (Frank and Pasquini, 2010). The Authors argue that ETTA allows reaching tuberculum sellae meningiomas through a direct and extracerebral approach, minimizing brain manipulation. Furthermore, it permits a frontal exposure of the anatomic regions that are not easy to visualize through intracranial approaches. However, ETTA has two main limits: 1) reduced versatility, and 2) the risk of cerebrospinal fluid leak. The cerebrospinal fluid leak is extremely variable. To prevent this complication, the Authors suggest the use of a multilayer autologous repair, but they also fell that, independently of the used technique, the range of post-operative cerebrospinal fluid leak can decrease only with an increased experience of surgeon, making the risk of the ETTA acceptable. Recently, advances in transsphenoidal endoscopic surgery have allowed difficult clival and petroclival tumors such as meningiomas causing effacement of the pons and basilar artery to be approached by this technique (Alexander et al., 2010). In past years, these meningiomas could be removed only with a transcranial approach. Now advances in transsphenoidal endoscopic surgery have allowed treatment of these tumors. The most common complications after a transsphenoidal approach are represented by meningitis, tension pneumocephalus and cerebrospinal fluid leak. Meningitis are directly associated with the incidence of untreated post-operative cerebrospinal fluid leak and range from 0,5% to 14%. Tension pneumocephalus has an incidence of less than 0,5%. The last but not the least complication is represented by postoperative cerebrospinal fluid leak, requiring a watertight dural closure, especially when surgeon needs to remove larger meningiomas. There are 4 ways to achieve the same goal: autografts and synthetic grafts; dural suturing with or without dural substitute; vascularized mucoseptal flap method; and the multilayer method. Those methods can be used singly or in combination (Saeki et al., 2010). In past years, lumbar drainage was often used to decrease intracranial pressure, facilitating closure of the dura mater; now the introduction in surgical practice of different types of grafts and sealant has rendered not routinely the use of a lumbar drainage (Kassam et al., 2005). Recenty, some Authors have described their opinion about different duraplasties, to establish the better way to prevent post-operative cerebrospinal fluid leak (Liu et al., 2011). Based on their own experience, they place intradurally an autologous fascia lata graft, holding it in place with several pieces of an absorbable haemostatic agent; next they tuck a layer of thick implantable acellular dermal graft at least 1 cm circumferentially between the remaining dural cuff and the edge of the bony defect; then bilateral mucosal flap pedicled on the posterior nasal artery are rotated over the acellular dermal graft to cover cranial base defects. Finally a thin layer of surgical sealant is placed over the multilayer closure (Germani et al., 2007); however, he did not use the flap and showed a postoperative cerebrospinal fluid leak range of 3%. With innovation made by Liu at al., they demonstrate a decrease in postoperative cerebrospinal fluid leak; moreover, mucosal flap, used as an additional layer, promotes rapid ingrowth of granulation, vascularization and re-epithelialization by sinonasal mucosa and allows surgeon to repair large skull base defects extending anteriorly to the posterior wall of the frontal sinus. On the other hand, some Authors have recently conducted a study on the use of equine collagen foil as dura mater substitute in endoscopic endonasal transsphenoidal surgery (Cappabianca et al., 2006). When an intraoperative cerebrospinal fluid leak is not demonstrated, they put the graft in place by the sole fibrin sealant that seems to be sufficient to prevent a postoperative cerebrospinal fluid leak. On the other hand, large intraoperative cerebrospinal fluid leak needs a multilayer dural reconstruction: the first layer of collagen matrix is put intradurally; the next step is the use of a solid or semisolid buttress to hold the sealing tissue in position and maintain the watertight seal to resist the pulsations of the brain and cerebrospinal fluid; then collagen sponges are put in the sphenoid sinus and, finally, fibrin glue is applied to ensure a watertight closure. Using this technique, Authors have demonstrated a post-operative cerebrospinal fluid leak range of 6,7%.

7. Complications of duraplasties

Cerebral or cerebellar swelling and shrinking margins of the dura mater during prolonged neurosurgery often necessitate a duraplasty to obtain a satisfactory watertight closure. However, despite the use of grafts, duraplasty are sometimes followed in post-operative observation by cerebrospinal fluid leakage, deep wound infection, asymptomatic pseudomeningocele, bleeding and hematomas, adherence formation, cerebral herniation, hypertensive pneumocephalus, epilepsy, chemical or bacterial meningitis, all resulting in a longer hospitalization.

Several complications are demonstrated after posterior fossa surgery. However, a well-performed duraplasty using a collagen matrix is safe and effective in the posterior fossa (Narotam et al., 2009). Authors have compared data derived from their experience with those represented in literature. Previous reports concerning posterior fossa dural repair using watertight seals demonstrate an average cerebrospinal fluid leakage rate of 7,7%, an average infection rate of 7,5%, an average asymptomatic pseudomeningocele, diagnosed with MRI and/or CT scan, rate of 11,8%. Using porous collagen matrix, Authors have found an average infection rate of 1,9% and an average asymptomatic pseudomeningocele rate of 3,8%; no cerebrospinal fluid leaks are described, so they argue that watertight dural closure is not essential in posterior fossa surgery.

Although rarer than posterior fossa surgery, complication are also frequent in sovratentorial approaches. Other Authors demonstrate an average infection rate of 4,5% using porous collagen matrix (Gnanalingham et al., 2002). Collagen matrix is used to obtain a watertight dural closure (Stendel et al., 2008); they report an average infection rate of 2,6%, an average cerebrospinal fluid leakage rate of 5,2% and an average cerebrospinal fluid fistula of 2,6%. Comparing this data with those obtained from literature, they have demonstrated that the use of collagen matrix determines a lower risk of infection and cerebrospinal fluid loss than the use of autograft or synthetic material. Moreover, postoperative infection seems to increase the risk of postoperative cerebrospinal fluid leakage.

Recently, the transmigration of fibrino-purulent and malignant cells into a dural graft was described (El Majdoub et al., 2008); this dural substitute is created with a non-absorbable, finely fibrillary, microporous, non-woven material of high purity aliphatic polyester urethane. Authors argue that local inflammation could create a local immunosuppression; moreover, the graft's implantation itself stimulates IL-10 and/or TGF- β secretion, enhancing immunosuppression and malignant cells infiltration of the graft.

Moreover, other Authors have recently reviewed literature about duraplasty in meningioma surgery and its related complication (Sade et al., 2011). The incidence of cerebrospinal fluid leakage reported in the literature varies, even when surgeons are using similar materials, probably indicating user-dependent variations. Authors demonstrate an average rate of 2 - 2,2% using acellular human dermis, an average rate of 15 % using allogenic cadaveric dura mater, an average rate of 3 % using allogenic and xenogenic pericardium and dura mater, an average rate of 10 % using autologous fascia, an average rate of 7 % using vicryl mesh, an average rate of 3 % using polytetrafluoroethylene and surgical sealant and an average rate of 20,3 % using polytetrafluoroethylene (alone). Other Authors have also published their own data about post-operative cerebrospinal fluid leak in a series of 128 patients who underwent posterior fossa surgery and in whom different types of duraplasty techniques and materials were used (Moskowitz et al., 2009): 25% using suturable bovine collagen, 12% with reformulated bovine collagen, 8% with acellular human dermis; no cerebrospinal fluid leak depending on the type of graft used are been demonstrated using bovine collagen matrix.

Inflammatory reactions can present in a time frame of 1–6 months following surgery; one of these complication is represented by chemical meningitis, that in general are more frequent in posterior fossa craniotomies (Forgacs et al., 2001) but this may not be applicable when it comes to chemical meningitis caused by a dural substitute. The incidence of chemical meningitis is 2,3% (Parizek et al., 1997). A higher incidence of inflammatory reactions was found after posterior fossa surgery (5,2%) compared with supratentorial locations (2%) (Sade et al., 2011); however, Authors emphasize that these data did not reach statistical significance.

The last but not the least problem related with dural reconstruction is represented by bacterial meningitis, a serious postoperative complication that can occur after the implantation of a foreign material. The incidences of postoperative infection differ in various studies, based on the use of various dural grafts (Sade et al., 2011): 1,5 - 2,2% using acellular human dermis, 0,6 % using allogenic and xenogenic fascia latae, pericardium and dura mater, 3,6 - 6,7% using collagen matrix and 9,6 % with polytetrafluoroethylene.

8. Future trends

Several searches of procedures and materials increase the contributions to the current debate on dural reconstruction. There are various schools of thought when it comes to dural reconstruction following meningioma surgery, which are largely based on the personal experience of the individual surgeons. Many schools perform preliminary evaluation of dura mater substitutes in the animals; with continued advances in chemical technology, it is inevitable that newer dural substitutes will be synthesized and they will be even closer to the normal dura, in terms of minimum or no inflammatory response, good handling characteristic, and biodegradability. Many dural substitutes have been tested in animals but not in humans; others, although used in human, have not been used long enough to assess the long-term results.

Some Authors have described a biodegradable elastic-fibrin material that is being used in humans; preliminary results have indicated that this material seems promising. In an experimental setting, the biodegradable elastin fibrin material produces minimal but histologically detectable inflammatory reaction; it is attenuated if a 0,2 mm thick graft is used rather than a 1 mm thick graft (San-Galli et al., 1996). Other Authors reported the use of biosynthetic cellulose as a dural substitute; they affirmed that the physical properties of biosynthetic cellulose and the low cellular reaction to its implantation qualify this material as an ideal dural substitute; like other materials, the use in humans is pending although experimental results are promising (Mello et al., 1997). Others described the use of hydroxylmethlmethacrylate hydrogels as potential dural substitute; experimental studies of this material have been promising, but the use in human is pending (Bathia et al., 1995). Others have developed a composite sheet composed of two layers of L-lactic acid ε-caprolactone with polyglycolic acid nonwoven fabric sandwiched between the layers. Clinical trials of this material are pending (Yamada et al., 1997). The vicryl mesh as a suitable dural substitute, with potential advantages, was performed to avoid cerebrospinal fluid leak, following posterior fossa surgery (Verheggen et al., 1997). Many methods to prevent postoperative cerebrospinal fluid leakage are available, but pressure-tight dural closure remains difficult, especially with synthetic surgical membranes. Other Authors assessed the efficacy of a novel dural closure technique, using absorbable polyglactin acid sheet and fibrin glue. They evaluated the results by detecting extradural or subcutaneous cerebrospinal fluid leakage on magnetic resonance imaging. They concluded that the combination of polyglactin acid sheet and fibrin glue can achieve watertight closure after intradural surgery and can minimize the risk of intractable postoperative cerebrospinal fluid leakage. But this simple, economical technique is recommended for dural closure after spinal intradural surgery (Sugawaraet al., 2005).

Some Authors compared cranial dural adhesions in a canine model, after duraplasty using nonpenetrating clips or penetrating needles and sutures. They concluded that duraplasties with clips displayed significantly less extensive acute and chronic inflammation, foreign body reaction, and meningoneural adherence than did repairs with needles and sutures (Palm et al., 1999).

Also about BioGlue there are innovative reports; this glue was applied as a reinforcement over collagen sponge as the last layer of the duraplasty. Authors concluded that this glue appears to be an effective adjunct in preventing postoperative cerebrospinal fluid leaks after transsphenoidal surgery. However, careful attention to technical details of the repair is still required to prevent failures, especially when closing large dural and diaphragmatic defects (Dusick et al., 2006). But the adequate repair of intraoperative cerebrospinal fluid leaks during transsphenoidal surgery remains a challenge. Other Authors have described the application of N-butyl 2-cyanoacrylate (cyanoacrylate) tissue glue for repair of cerebrospinal fluid fistulas during transsphenoidal surgery; they concluded that this glue appears to be effective and safe in preventing postoperative cerebrospinal fluid leakage (Cohen-Gadol et al., 2010).

Recently, a new polyethylene glycol dural sealant product was reported as effective at preventing cerebrospinal fluid leak after posterior fossa surgery (Than et al., 2008). Another technique for minor dural gap repair was reported; these Authors performed the duraplasty with a piece of oxidized cellulose, reinforced by fibrin glue, as a sutureless graft with more ease and less technical demand than other techniques. This procedure is a fast and valid alternative to small dural defect closure methods (Gazzeri et al., 2011).

All experimental and clinical studies consider new procedures or new materials, but the newer search field is dural cell colture. Some Authors have analyzed the dural cell culture as a new approach to achieve a duraplasty. Their study succeeded in establishing a cell culture model for duraplasty and indicated cellular migration from the dura borders at the site of the defect during the wound healing process. The cell culture model presented in this report shows that collagen grafts are best suited for duraplasty. In accordance with the immunocytological finding of fibroblast migration from the dura borders, additional application of fibroblast-stimulating growth factors accelerated cellular defect closure (Schick et al., 2003). Other Authors affirmed that fibrin glue is an attractive extracellular matrix for cellular migration from the dura, which is suited to fibroblast culturing in suture nets. Their findings supported the idea of achieving closure of cerebrospinal fluid fistulas by suture application of autologous fibroblasts and fibrin/thrombin preparations as a realistic future goal (Wolf et al., 2005). Also another study have demonstrated that an in vitro model for dural healing was successfully constructed in collagen-coated wells; results implicate cellular migration of fibroblasts from the dural defect margin as an important mechanism of wound healing following duraplasty (Zhou et al., 2006). These evaluations confirm our clinical observations about our cases of duraplasty. On the other hand, there are many searches about mesenchymal stem cells; some Authors have assessed the ability of rat bone marrow derived mesenchymal stem cells, in the presence of a growth factor, (fibroblast growth factor-4 and hydroxyapatite), to act as a scaffold for posterolateral spinal fusion in a rat model (Seo et al., 2009). Recently, human embryonic stem cell-derived mesenchymal cells were described, investigating the efficacy of these cells for cardiac repair after myocardial infarction (Simpson et al., 2011). Finally, the tissue engineering of multilayered constructs that model complex tissues poses a significant challenge for regenerative medicine. Some Authors have reported a three-layered scaffold consisting of an electrospun silk fibroin mat sandwiched between two dense collagen layers, providing an extracellular matrix-like environment for mesenchymal stem cells. They concluded that the ease of multilayered construct fabrication, enhanced biomechanical properties, along with uniformity of cell distribution confirmed the possibility for the incorporation and segregation of different cell types within distinct layers for the regeneration of complex tissues, such as skin, or central nervous system dura mater (Ghezzi et al., 2011). In the foreseeable future, several promising procedures and several synthetically derived dural substitute may be avaible for human use that contain most of the attributes of an ideal dural substitute.

9. References

Alexander, H.; Robinson, S.; Wickremesekera, A. & Wormald, P.J. (2010). Endoscopic transsphenoidal resection of a mid-clival meningioma. Journal of Clinical Neuroscience, Vol.17, No.3, (March 2010), pp. 374–376.

Bassiouni, H.; Asgari, S. & Stolke, D. (2006). Tuberculum sellae meningiomas: functional outcome in a consecutive series treated microsurgically. Surgical Neurology, Vol.66, No.1, (July 2006), pp. 37–44.

Bhatia, S.; Bergethon, P.R.; Blease, S.; Kemper, T.; Rosiello, A.; Zimbardi, G.P.; Franzblau, C. & Spatz, E.L. (1995). A synthetic dural prosthesis constructed from hydroxyethylmethacrylate hydrogels. Journal of Neurosurgery, Vol.83, No.5, (November 1995), pp. 897-902.

Biroli, F.; Fusco, M.; Bani, G.G.; Signorelli, A.; Esposito, F.; de Divitiis, O.; Cappabianca, P.; Cavallo, L.M. (2008). Novel equine collagen-only dural substitute. Neurosurgery, Vol.62, No.3 Suppl.1, (March 2008), pp. 273–274.

Black, P. (2000). Cerebrospinal fluid leaks following spinal or posterior fossa surgery: use of fat grafts for prevention and repair. Neurosurgical Focus, Vol.9, No.1, (July 2000).

Cappabianca, P.; Esposito, F.; Cavallo, L.M.; Messina, A.; Solari, D.; di Somma, L.G.M. & de Divitiis, E. (2006). Use of equine collagen foil as dura mater substitute in endoscopic endonasal transsphenoidal surgery. Surgical Neurology, Vol.65, No.2, (February 2006), pp. 144–149.

Caroli, E.; Rocchi, G.; Salvati, M. & Delfini R. (2004). Duraplasty: Our Current Experience. Surgical Neurology, Vol.61, No.1, (January 2004), pp. 55–59.

Chaplin, J.M.; Costantino, P.D.; Wolpoe, M.E.; Bederson, J.B.; Griffey, E. & Zanh, W.X. (1999). Use of Acellular dermal allograft for dural replacement: an experimental study. Neurosurgery, Vol.45, No.2, (August 1999), pp. 320–327.

Chappell, E.T.; Pare, L.; Salehpour, M.; Mathews, M. & Middlehof, C. (2009). GORE PRECLUDE MVP dura substitute applied as a nonwatertight "underlay" graft for craniotomies: product and technique evaluation. Surgical Neurology, Vol.71, No.1, (January 2009), pp. 126–129.

Cohen-Gadol, A.A.; Bellew, M.P.; Akard, W. & Payner, T.D. (2010). The application of n-butyl 2-cyanoacrylate to repair CSF fistulas for 221 patients who underwent transsphenoidal surgery. Minimally Invasive Neurosurgery, Vol.53, No.4, (August 2010), pp. 207-209.

Cosgrove, G.R.; Delashaw, J.B.; Grotenhuis, J.A.; Tew, J.M.; Van Loveren, H.; Spetzler, R.F.; Payner, T.; Rosseau, G.; Shaffrey, M.E.; Hopkins, L.N.; Byrne, R. & Norbash, A. (2007). Safety and efficacy of a novel polyethylene glycol hydrogel sealant for watertight dural repair. Journal of Neurosurgery, Vol.106, No.1, (January 2007), pp. 52–58.

Dusick, J.R.; Mattozo, C.A.; Esposito, F. & Kelly, D.F. (2006). BioGlue for prevention of postoperative cerebrospinal fluid leaks in transsphenoidal surgery: A case series. Surgical Neurology, Vol.66, No.4, (October 2006), pp. 371-376.

El Majdoub, F.; Lohr, M.; Maarouf, M.; Brunn, A.; Stenzel, W. & Ernestus, R.I. (2009). Transmigration of fibrino-purulent inflammation and malignant cells into an artificial dura substitute (Neuro-Patch): report of two cases. Acta Neurochirurgica, Vol.151, No.7, (July 2009), pp. 833–835.

Epstein N.E. (2010). Dural repair with four spinal sealants: focused review of the manufacturers' inserts and the current literature. The Spine Journal, Vol.10, No.12, (December 2010), pp. 1065–1068.

Forgacs, P.; Geyer, C.A. & Freidberg, S.R. (2001). Characterization of chemical meningitis after neurological surgery. Clinical Infectious Disease, Vol.32, No.2, (January 2001), pp. 179–185.

Frank, G. & Pasquini, E. (2010). Tuberculum Sellae Meningioma: The Extended Transsphenoidal Approach - For the Virtuoso Only? World Neurosurgery, Vol.73, No.6, (June 2010), pp. 625–626.

Gazzeri, R.; Neroni, M.; Alfieri, A.; Galarza, M.; Faiola, A.; Esposito, S. & Giordano, M. (2009). Transparent equine collagen biomatrix as dural repair. A prospective clinical study. Acta Neurochirurgica, Vol.151, No.5, (May 2009), pp. 537–543.

Gazzeri, R.; Galarza, M.; Alfieri, A.; Neroni, M. & Roperto R. (2011). Simple intraoperative technique for minor dural gap repair using fibrin glue and oxidized cellulose. World Neurosurgery, Vol.76, No.1-2, (July-August 2011), pp. 173-175.

Germani, R.M.; Vivero, R.; Herzallah, I.R. & Casiano, R.R. (2007). Endoscopic reconstruction of large anterior skull base defects using acellular dermal allograft. American Journal of Rhinology, Vol.21, No.5, (September-October 2007), pp. 615–618.

Ghezzi, C.E.; Marelli, B.; Muja, N.; Hirota, N.; Martin, J.G.; Barralet, J.E.; Alessandrino, A.; Freddi, G. & Nazhat, S.N. (2011). Mesenchymal stem cell-seeded multilayered dense collagen-silk fibroin hybrid for tissue engineering applications. Biotechnology Journal, doi: 10.1002/biot.201100127.

Gnanalingham, K.K.; Lafuente, J.; Thompson, D.; Harkness, W. & Hayward, R. (2002). Surgical procedures for posterior fossa tumors in children: does craniotomy lead to fewer complications than craniectomy? Journal of Neurosurgery, Vol.97, No.4, (October 2002), pp. 821–826.

Hida, K.; Yamaguchi, S.; Seki, T.; Yano, S.; Akino, M.; Terasaka, S.; Uchida, T. & Iwasaki, Y. (2006). Nonsuture dural repair using polyglycolic acid mesh and fibrin glue: clinical application to spinal surgery. Surgical Neurology, Vol.65, No.2, (February 2006), pp. 136–142.

Hwang, P.H. & Jackler R.K. (1996). Lipoid meningitis due to aseptic necrosis of a free fat graft placed during neurotologic surgery. Laryngoscope, Vol.106, No.12 Pt.1, (December 1996), pp. 1482–1486.

Islam, S.; Ogane, K.; Ohkuma, H. & Suzuki, S. (2004). Usefulness of acellular dermal graft as a dural substitute in experimental model. Surgical Neurology, Vol.61, No. 3, (March 2004), pp. 297–302.

Ito, H.; Kimura, T.; Sameshima, T.; Aiyama, H.; Nishimura, K.; Ochiai, C. & Morita, A. (2011). Reinforcement of pericranium as a dural substitute by fibrin sealant. Acta Neurochirurgica, Vol.6, (July 2011).

Jallo, G.I. & Benjamin, V. (2002). Tuberculum sellae meningiomas: microsurgical anatomy and surgical technique. Neurosurgery, Vol.51, No.6, (December 2002), pp. 1432–1439.

Kassam, A.; Carrau, R.L. & Snyderman, C.H. (2005). Evolution of reconstructive techniques following endoscopic expanded endonasal approaches. Neurosurgical Focus, Vol.19, No.1, (July 2005).

Kim, D.W.; Eum, W.S.; Jang, S.H.; Park, J., Heo, D.H.; Sheen, S.H.; Lee, H.R.; Kweon, H.; Kang, S.W.; Lee, K.G.; Cho, S.Y.; Jin H.J.; Cho, Y.J. & Choi, S.Y. (2011). A transparent artificial dura mater made of silk fibroin as an inhibitor of inflammation in craniotomized rats. Journal of Neurosurgery, Vol. 114, No.2, (February 2011), pp. 485–490.

Knopp, U.; Christmann, F.; Reusche, E. & Sepehrnia, A. (2005). A new collagen biomatrix of equine origin versus a cadaveric dura graft for the repair of dural defects–a comparative animal experimental study. Acta Neurochirurgica, Vol.147, No.8, (August 2005), pp. 877–887.

Lee, J.H. (2008). Meningiomas, Springer-Verlag, 978-1-84628-526-4, London.

Liu, J.K.; Christiano, L.D.; Patel, S.K.; Tubbs, S. & Eloy, J.A. *(2011).* Surgical nuances for removal of olfactory groove meningiomas using the endoscopic endonasal transcribriform approach. *Neurosurgical Focus, Vol.30, No.5, (May 2011), E3.*

McAllister, J.D.; Scotti, L.N. & Bookwalter, J.W. (1992). Postoperative dissemination of fat particles in the subarachnoid pathways. American Journal of Neuroradiology, Vol.13, No.4, (July-August 1992), pp. 1265–1267.

Megyesi, J.F.; Ranger, A.; MacDonald, W. & Del Maestro, R.F. (2004). Suturing technique and the integrity of dural closures: an in vitro study. Neurosurgery, Vol.55, No.4, (October 2004), pp. 950–954.

Mello, L.R.; Feltrin, L.T.; Fontes Neto, P.T. & Ferraz, F.A. (1997). Duraplasty with biosynthetic cellulose: an experimental study. Journal of Neurosurgery, Vol.86, No.1, (January 1997), pp. 143-150.

Moskowitz, S.I.; Liu, J. & Krishnaney, A.A. (2009). Postoperative complications associated with dural substitutes in suboccipital craniotomies. Neurosurgery, Vol.64, No.3 Suppl., (March 2009), pp. 28–34.

Narotam, P.K.; van Dellen, J.R. & Bhoola, K.D. (1995). A clinicopathological study of collagen sponge as a dural graft in neurosurgery. Journal of Neurosurgery, Vol. 82, No.3, (March 1995), pp. 406–412.

Narotam, P.K.; Reddy, K.; Fewer, D.; Qiao, F. & Nathoo, N. (2007) Collagen matrix duraplasty for cranial and spinal surgery: a clinical and imaging study. Journal of Neurosurgery, Vol.106, No.1, (January 2007), pp. 45–51.

Narotam, P.K.; Qiao, F. & Nathoo, N. (2009). Collagen matrix duraplasty for posterior fossa surgery: evaluation of surgical technique in 52 adult patients. Journal of Neurosurgery, Vol.111, No.2, (August 2009), pp. 380–386.

Palm, S.J.; Kirsch, W.M.; Zhu, Y.H.; Peckham, N.; Kihara, S.; Anton, R.; Anton, T.; Balzer, K. & Eickmann, T. (1999). Dural closure with nonpenetrating clips prevents meningoneural adhesions: an experimental study in dogs. Neurosurgery, Vol.45, No.4, (October 1999), pp. 881-882.

Parizek, J.; Měricka, P.; Husek, Z.; Suba, P.; Spacek, J. & Nomecek, S. (1997). Detailed evaluation of 2959 allogeneic and xenogeneic dense connective tissue grafts (fascia lata, pericardium, and dura mater) used in the course of 20 years for duraplasty in neurosurgery. Acta Neurochirurgica, Vol.139, No.9, pp. 827–838.

Parlato, C.; di Nuzzo, G.; Luongo, M.; Parlato, R.S.; Accardo, M.; Cuccurullo, L.; Moraci, A. (2011). Use of a collagen biomatrix (TissuDura) for dura repair: a long-term neuroradiological and neuropathological evaluation. Acta Neurochirurgica, Vol.153, No.1, (January 2011), pp. 142–147.

Protasoni, M.; Sangiorgi, S.; Cividini, A.; Culuvaris, G.T.; Tomei, G.; Dell'Orbo, C.; Raspanti, M.; Balbi, S. & Reguzzoni, M. (2011). The collagenic architecture of human dura mater. Journal of Neurosurgery, Vol.114, No.6, (June 2011), pp. 1723–1730.

Reddy, M.; Schoggl, A.; Reddy, B.; Saringer, W.; Weigel, G. & Matula, C. (2002). A Clinical Study of a Fibrinogen-Based Collagen Fleece for Dural Repair in Neurosurgery. Acta Neurochirurgica, Vol.144, No.3, (March 2002), pp. 265–269.

Ricaurte, J.C.; Murali, R. & Mandell, W. (2000). Uncomplicated postoperative lipoid meningitis secondary to autologous fat graft necrosis. Clinical Infectious Disease, Vol.30, No.3, (March 2000), pp. 613–615.

Sade, B.; Oya, S. & Lee, J.H. (2011). Non-watertight dural reconstruction in meningioma surgery: results in 439 consecutive patients and a review of the literature. Journal of Neurosurgery, Vol.114, No.3, (March 2011), pp. 714–718.

Saeki, N.; Horiguchi, K.; Murai, H.; Hasegawa, Y.; Hanazawa, T. & Okamoto, Y. (2010). Endoscopic endonasal pituitary and skull base surgery. Neurologia Medico-Chirurgica (Tokyo), Vol.50, No.9, pp. 756–764.

San-Galli, F.; Deminiere, C.; Guerin, J. & Rabaud M. (1996). Use of a biodegradable elastin-fibrin material, Neoplast, as a dural substitute. Biomaterials, Vol.17, No.11, (June 1996), pp. 1081-1085.

Schick, B.; Wolf, G.; Romeike, B.F.; Mestres, P.; Praetorius, M. & Plinkert, P.K. (2003). Dural cell culture. A new approach to study duraplasty. Cells Tissues Organs, Vol.173, No.3, pp. 129-137.

Seo, H.S.; Jung, J.K.; Lim, M.H.; Hyun, D.K.; Oh, N.S. & Yoon, S.H. (2009). Evaluation of Spinal Fusion Using Bone Marrow Derived Mesenchymal Stem Cells with or without Fibroblast Growth Factor-4. Journal of Korean Neurosurgical Society, Vol.46, No.4, pp. 397-402.

Simpson, D.L.; Boyd, N.L.; Kaushal, S.; Stice, S.L. & Dudley, S.C. Jr. (2011). Use of human embryonic stem cell derived-mesenchymal cells for cardiac repair. Biotechnology and Bioengineering, doi: 10.1002/bit.23301.

Stendel, R.; Danne, M.; Fiss, I.; Klein, I.; Schilling, A.; Hammersen, S.; Pietilae, T.; Janisch, W. & Hopfenmuller, W. (2008). Efficacy and safety of a collagen matrix for cranial and spinal dural reconstruction using different fixation techniques. Journal of Neurosurgery, Vol.109, No.2, (August 2008), pp. 215–221.

Sugawara, T.; Itoh, Y.; Hirano, Y.; Higashiyama, N.; Shimada, Y.; Kinouchi, H. & Mizoi, K. (2005). Novel dural closure technique using polyglactin acid sheet prevents cerebrospinal fluid leakage after spinal surgery. Neurosurgery, Vol.57, No.4 Suppl, (October 2005), pp. 290-294.

Taha, A.N.; Almefty, R.; Pravdenkova, S. & Al-Mefty, O. (2011). Sequelae of Autologous Fat Graft Used for Reconstruction in Skull Base Surgery. World Neurosurgery, Vol.75, No.5-6, (May-June 2011), pp. 692–695.

Than, K.D.; Baird, C.J. & Olivi, A. (2008). Polyethylene glycol hydrogel dural sealant may reduce incisional cerebrospinal fluid leak after posterior fossa surgery. Neurosurgery, Vol. 63, No.1, (July 2008), pp. 186-187.

Verheggen, R.; Schulte-Baumann, W.J.; Hahm, G.; Lang, J.; Freudenthaler, S.; Schaake, T. & Markakis, E. (1997). A new technique of dural closure--experience with a vicryl mesh. Acta Neurochirurgica, Vol.139, No.11, pp. 1074-1079.

Wang, Q.; Lu, X.J.; Ji1, W.Y.; Yan, Z.C.; Xu, J.; Ding, Y.S. & Zhang, J. (2010). Visual Outcome After Extended Endoscopic Endonasal Transsphenoidal Surgery for Tuberculum Sellae Meningiomas. World Neurosurgery, Vol.73, No.6, (June 2010), pp. 694–700.

Warren, W.L.; Medary, M.B.; Dureza, C.D.; Bellotte, J.B.; Flannagan, P.P.; Oh, M.Y. & Fukushima, T. (2000). Dural repair using acellular human dermis: experience with 200 cases: technique assessment. Neurosurgery, Vol.46, No.6, (June 2000), pp. 1391–1396.

Wolf, G.; Plinkert, P.K. & Schick, B. (2005). Cell transplantation for a CSF-fistula. Experience with fibrin glue and fibroblasts. HNO, Vol.53, No.5, pp. 439-445.

Yamada, K.; Miyamoto, S.; Nagata, I.; Kikuchi, H.; Ikada, Y.; Iwata, H. & Yamamoto, K. (1997). Development of a dural substitute from synthetic bioabsorbable polymers. Journal of Neurosurgery, Vol.86, No.6, (June 1997), pp. 1012–1017.

Zhou, F.; Chen, G.; Zhang, J.M. & Huang, Z.S. (2006). An in vitro culturing model for rabbit dural cells. Annals of Clinical and Laboratory Science, Vol.36, No.3, pp. 341-344.

7

Surgical Approaches for Lateral Ventricular Trigone Meningioma

Takafumi Nishizaki
Department of Neurosurgery, Ube Industries Central Hospital, Japan

1. Introduction

Intraventricular meningiomas account for 9.8-14% of all intraventricular tumors and for 20% of lateral ventricle tumors [1,2]. Meningiomas of the lateral ventricle constitute 0.5-4.5% of all intracranial meningiomas [3,4]. Between 60% and 94% of them arise from the choroid plexus at the trigone. The predilection for the trigone may be attributed to the abundance of choroid plexus arachnoidea. The clinical manifestations of lateral ventricular meningiomas depend on the tumor size [5]: A small tumor causes no clinical symptoms because the lateral ventricle has a relatively large compensating space. The most common initial symptoms are headaches, vomiting and consciousness disturbance related to increased intracranial pressure. Sensori-motor deficits, clumsiness, ataxia, and cognitive impairment including dysphasia, dyslexia, dysgraphia, and dyscalcula, are sometimes observed according to the tumor location. Visual field deficits and seizures are present, especially in patients with large tumors. Other unusual symptoms, such as epilepsy, can also occur [6]. Cushing and Eisenhardt grouped the symptoms caused by large ventricular meningiomas into the following types [7]: (a) headache caused by increased intracranial pressure; (b) contralateral spotted homonymous hemianopsia; (c) contralateral sensory disturbance and hemiparesis; (d) symptoms of cerebellar damage; and (e) possible paralexia in patients with tumors located on the left side.

The radiological appearance of intraventricular meningiomas is similar to those at other locations. CT and MRI demonstrate the tumors as a well-defined mass. Most tumors display homogeneous and strong enhancement with contrast medium. Perifocal edema is evident, and minimal to massive calcifications are present in 47% of cases [4,8,910,11]). Hydrocephalus or a trapped occipital horn can be observed in patients with large tumors. Angiography shows the tumors to be supplied by both the anterior and posterior choroidal arteries, or by the posterior choroidal arteries only. The cisternal and initial ventricular segment is pushed down and forward by the enlarging temporal horn. The blood supply is predominantly from the anterior choroidal artery, and large tumors receive a significant supply from posterior choroidal artery. Intraventricular meningiomas show the characteristic histological appearance of meningioma. Bertalanffy et al. reported that the majority (75%) of such tumors were of the meningothelial or mixed type, and that 19% were atypical.

2. Surgical approach

Surgical approaches for trigone meningioma is challenging, because excessive cortical dissection or brain retraction carries a risk of post-operative visual field deficit, speech disturbance, or epilepsy. Occlusion of posterior and anterior choroidal blood supplies is also important to achieve tumor hemostasis. Thus, there is still a degree of controversy regarding the optimal surgical approach for this tumour. Several surgical approaches have been described for trigone meningiomas, each with their proponents (Figure1-A and B). In this chapter, recognised benefits and drawbacks of previously-reported approaches and the optimal approach for lateral ventricular trigone meningioma are discussed.

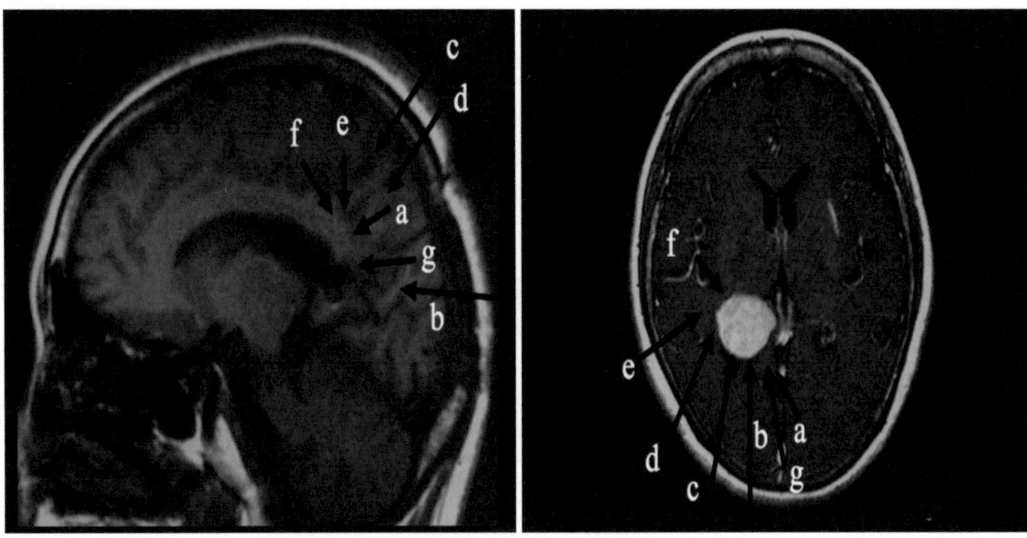

Fig. 1. (A: sagittal view, B: axial view) Surgical approaches devised for trigone meningiomas (a: occipital trans-callosal, b: lateral occipital, c: high parietal paramedian, d: inferior parietal, e: temporal horn, f: lateral trans-sulcal, g: occipital interhemispheric)

2.1 Occipital trans-callosal approach (Figure 1-a)

The trans-callosal approach is an appropriate choice for excision of third-ventricular lesions when the corpus callosum section is limited to the anterior two thirds of the body and the genu. Occipital craniotomy and a trans-callosal approach reduce the incidence of postoperative seizures, speech disturbance and visual field deficits [13], and facilitate early exposure of the posterior choroidal artery. This procedure can be performed without significant postsurgical deficits attributable to the disconnection procedure, especially for small trigonal tumors. The disadvantage of this approach is complete section of the splenium of the corpus callosum, which interrupts the transfer of cortical visual information from the non-dominant hemisphere to the speech centres. When right homonymous hemianopsia is associated with complete section, alexia without agraphia may occur. Also, preoperative right homonymous hemianopsia is a relative contraindication for the trans-callosal approach.

2.2 Lateral occipital approach (Figure 1-b)

Lateral occipital lobectomy can reduce the degree of cerebral retraction, although the vascular pedicles may not be easily accessible [14]. When the brain surface is incised near the angular gyrus, it can result in homonymous hemianopsia or alexia [15]. Use of this approach is limited to avascular tumors and patients with homonymous hemianopsia caused by relatively large tumors.

2.3 High parietal paramedian approach (Figure 1-c)

A high parietal paramedian incision usually extends from the postcentral to parieto-occipital fissure, approximately 3 cm from the falx, and lies medial to the majority of visual fibers, and running parallel to their projection [16]. A high parietal paramedian incision, which may avoid damage to the optic radiation or creation of a permanent speech deficit, sometimes causes motor weakness or seizures. However, Fornari et al. reported that although this approach caused no permanent motor or speech deficits, it preserved visual function in only 2 of 18 patients [9]. This approach can cause postoperative neurological deficits associated with parietal lobe function and visual-spatial processing. Apraxia and acalculia may occur in the dominant hemisphere. Another drawback of this approach is that it cannot provide early exposure of the feeding arteries.

2.4 Inferior parietal approach (Figure 1-d)

An inferior parietal incision minimising the depth of brain that needs to be traversed, brings the surgeons close to the tumor. However, homonymous hemianopsia can occur if the lateral aspect of the optic radiation is divided [17,18]. Manipulation of the angular gyrus in the dominant hemisphere also carries a risk of language impairment including agraphia, alexia, acalculia, and sometimes Gerstmann's syndrome. In the non-dominant hemisphere it jeopardises retention of visual information or spatial perception. Another serious drawback is that early exposure and hemostasis of the feeding arteries are difficult with this approach, and it is particularly contraindicated for highly vascular tumors.

2.5 Middle temporal and temporal horn approach (Figure 1-e)

A temporal horn approach through the middle temporal gyrus allows preliminary occlusion of the anterior choroidal artery [19]. This approach can minimize the depth of brain that needs to be traversed. Posoperative homonymous visual field impairment may occur, but damage to the optic radiation can be minimized if the incision is parallel to the optic fibers. However, it can cause speech and auditory comprehension deficits. Anomic aphasia can occur after excision of a meningioma in the dominant hemisphere via a middle temporal gyrus incision [19]. An anterior temporal horn and trigone approach via a more inferior temporo-occipital incision, lessening the degree of speech deficit [20], can cause a superior quadrant field defect. Damage to the dominant middle temporal gyrus may impair capabilities for reading, naming and phoneme identification [20]. The non-dominant middle temporal gyrus is associated with recognition of emotion. While the posterior choroidal artery is not visible until the majority of the tumor has been removed, early control of the anterior choroidal artery can be achieved. This approach can be a first choice for vascular meninigoma of the non-dominant hemisphere, fed mainly by the anterior choroidal artery.

2.6 Lateral trans-sulcal approach (Figure 1-f)

A lateral trans-sulcal approach involves opening of the posterior part of the sylvian fissure or superior temporal sulcus [21]. This approach through the former and latter has been adopted for patients with a wide and a narrow sylvian cistern, respectively, and can reduce the risk of morbidity even in the dominant ventricle by minimizing any damage to the temporal gyrus. Nagata et al. have reported that patients with meningiomas in the dominant hemisphere exhibited transient amnestic aphasia and dyscalculia postoperatively, but the symptoms disappeared in a few days or weeks [21].

2.7 Occipital interhemispheric subcortical approach (Figure 1-g)

This approach invariably minimises postoperative neurological deficits including any damage to the lateral aspect of the optic radiation or corpus callosum [22]

Patient position and extent of craniotomy: When this approach is performed with the patient in a sitting position, there has been significant concern about the risk of venous air embolism. Also, it is occasionally difficult to reach the para-splenial cisterns for release of cerebrospinal fluid (CSF). The occipital interhemispheric approach can be performed in the lateral semi-prone position (Figure 2). Positioning the head of the patient so that the tumour-containing ventricle is oriented downwards and laterally allows easy access to the para-splenial cisterns without risk of venous embolism. As the tumour-containing occipital lobe is pulled down by gravity, retraction of the medial surface of the hemisphere can be reduced. In most cases of meningioma, this approach does not require preoperative lumbar spinal drainage or intraoperative ventricular tap. Before the cortical incision, the arachnoid around the bridging veins entering the great vein of Galen should be dissected and safely released. Retraction becomes progressively easier as the tumour is debulked and cerebrospinal fluid is released from the ventricle, thus decreasing the risk to the visual cortex resulting from retraction. After releasing CSF from the para-splenial cistern, a brain retractor is used so as not to pull back the occipital lobe, but only to open the incised brain surface. Occipital craniotomy seems adequate for surgical manipulation of the tumour, because the occipital interhemispheric fissure often lacks important bridging veins in comparison with the parieto-occipital interhemispheric fissure.

Tumor landmark: The area of cortical incision is important for minimally invasive microsurgery. Intraoperative navigation to identify the tumours can allow easy access to the tumour surface (about 1 cm in depth) and minimise any brain damage. Ultrasonography can be used for tumor identification (Figure 3), and the great vein of Galen is a good landmark. Small tumours less than 2.5 cm in diameter can be removed via an incision less than 1.5 cm long.

Hemostasis of tumor vasculature: Most lateral trans-cortical and trans-sulcal approaches, except for the temporal horn approach, do not allow early access to the vascular pedicles, as blood supply is sparser in the lateral aspect of the tumour. This approach, allowing early exposure of the medial surface of the tumour without injury to the splenium, is as useful as the trans-callosal approach. The posterior and anterior choroidal blood supplies are usually from the posterior- and anterior-medial aspects of the tumour, respectively (Figure 4). Debulking of the medial part of the tumour first allows early control of the posterior, and then anterior, choroidal blood supplies to the lesion.

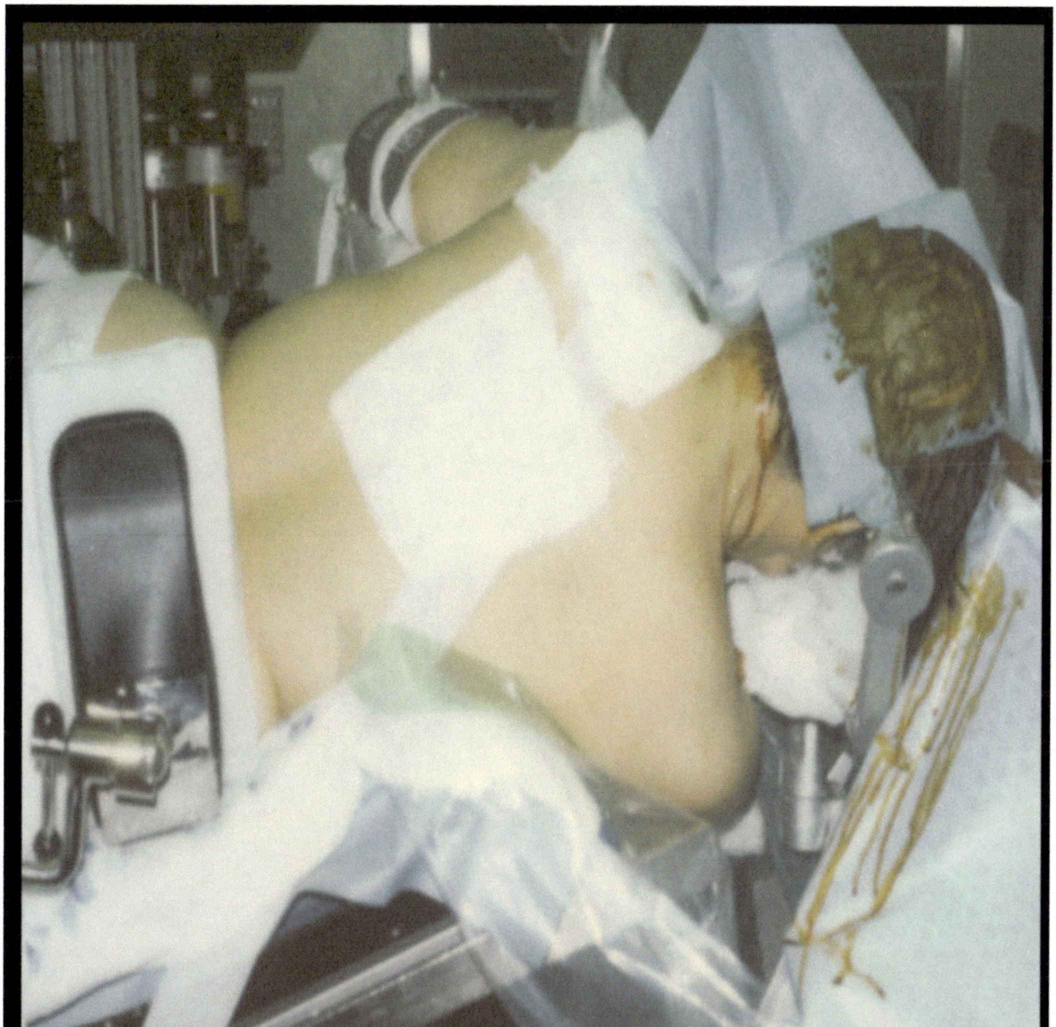

Fig. 2. Lateral semi-prone position, positioning the head of the patient so that the tumour-containing ventricle is oriented downwards and laterally

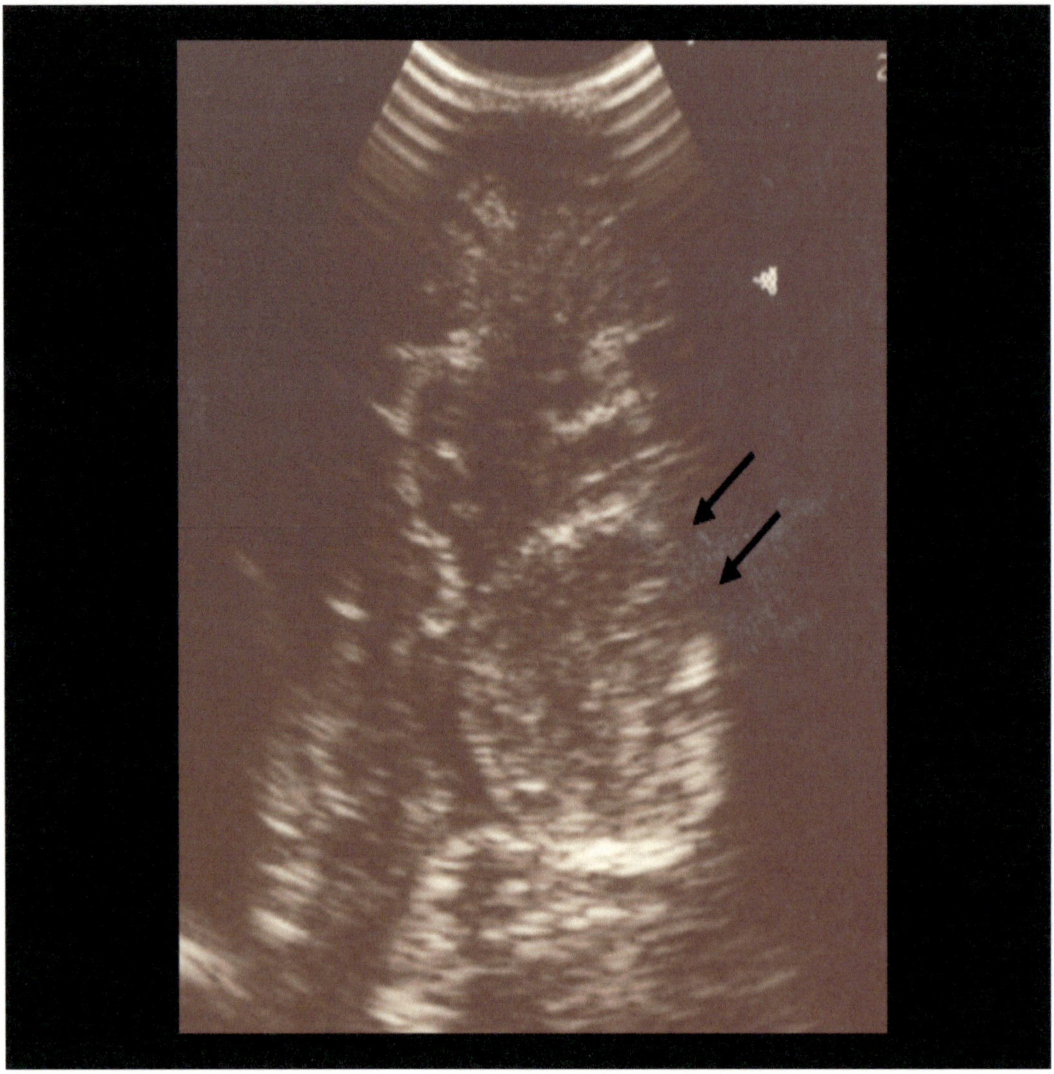

Fig. 3. Intraoperative ultrasonography used for tumor identification as well as intraoperative navigation (arrow: tumour contour)

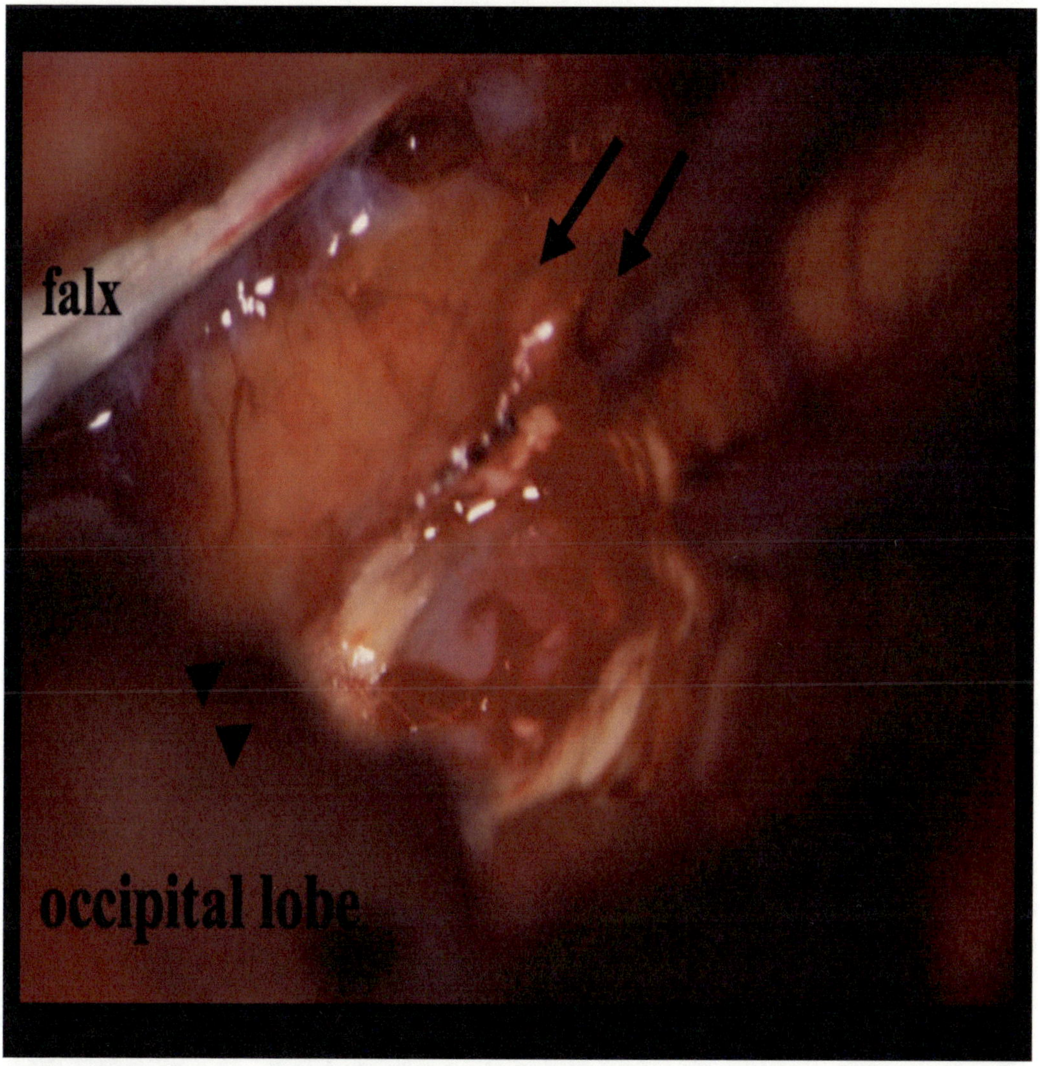

Fig. 4. Intraoperative view of the trigone meningioma. In cases of meningioma, the posterior and anterior choroidal blood supplies coming from the posterior- (arrowhead) and anterior-medial aspects (arrow) of the tumour, respectively.

Special remarks: Immediately after surgery, some patients have mild left-sided visual agnosia, but this resolves completely within one day after the operation. After surgery, there is a lower incidence of postoperative seizures, and no risk to speech function. One pitfall of this approach is possible transient memory disturbance in the dominant hemisphere. Special care must be taken so as not to injure the fornix, as this can cause permanent sequelae, even in cases where the tumour is located in the non-dominant hemisphere. Cognitive function should be carefully evaluated when this approach is adopted for a trigone meningioma in the dominant hemisphere. An occipital inter-hemispheric and transcortical approach with the patient in the lateral semiprone position is useful for decreasing the risk of post-operative hemianopia, epilepsy, or speech disturbance, even in patients with a tumour in the dominant hemisphere.

Similar approach to other brain tumors: The occipital interhemispheric approach has been used for pineal region tumors and tentorial meningioma (Figure 5). The occipital interhemispheric transcortical approach can be used in patients with occipital tumors (Figure 6) or other trigone tumors (Figure 7). Special attention must be paid to brain edema, especially in patients with malignant tumors (Figure 7). Immediate and direct approaches to the trigone for release of CSF, or preoperative CSF drainage, are sometimes necessary. The blood supply of a malignant tumor differs from that of meningioma. Unlike meningioma, malignant tumors tend to have the vascular pedicles as a blood supply over the whole tumor surface. Also, CSF dissemination can occur in cases of malignant tumor, because this procedure is performed via the ventricle.

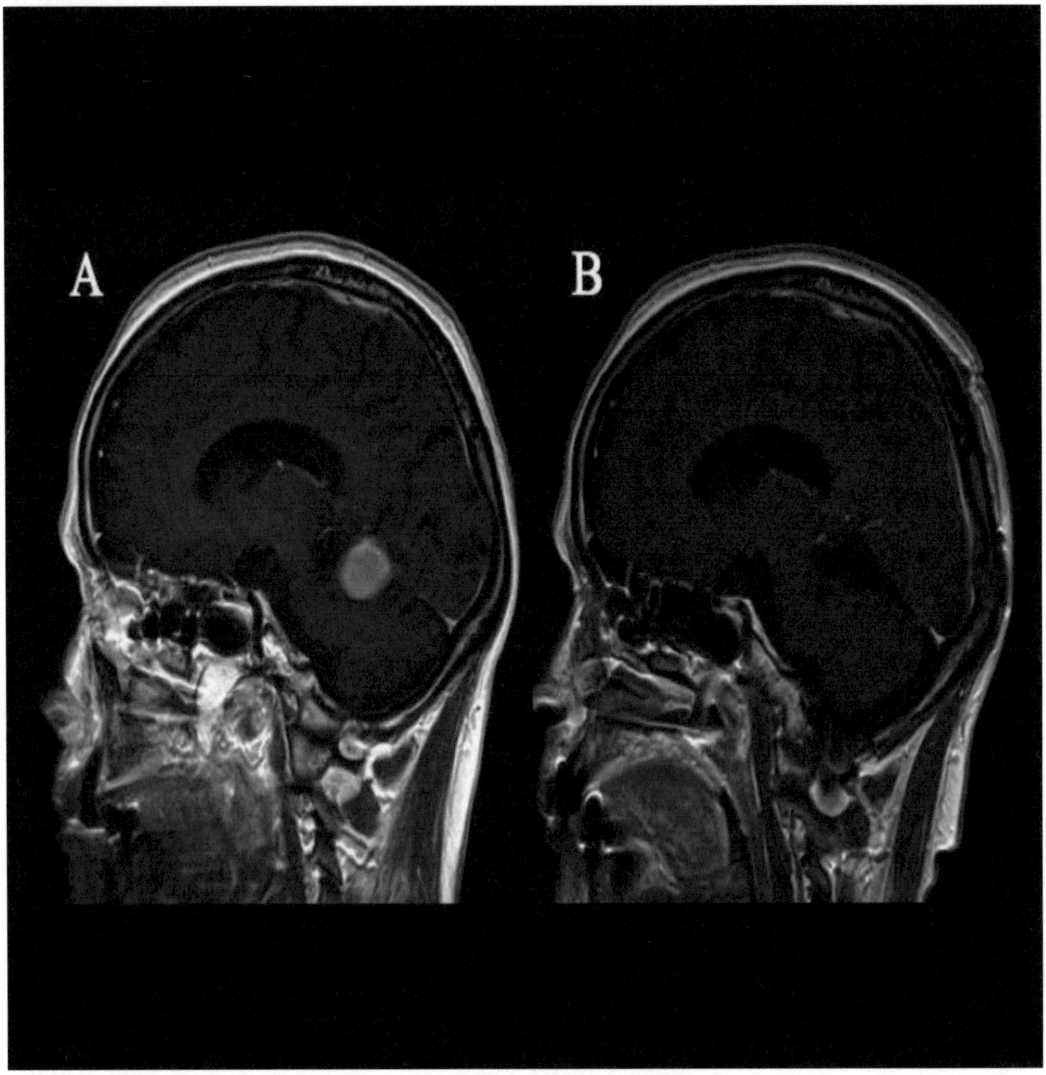

Fig. 5. tentorial meningioma. (A: preoperative MRI revealing left tentorial meningioma. B: postoperative MRI demonstrating total removal of the tumour)

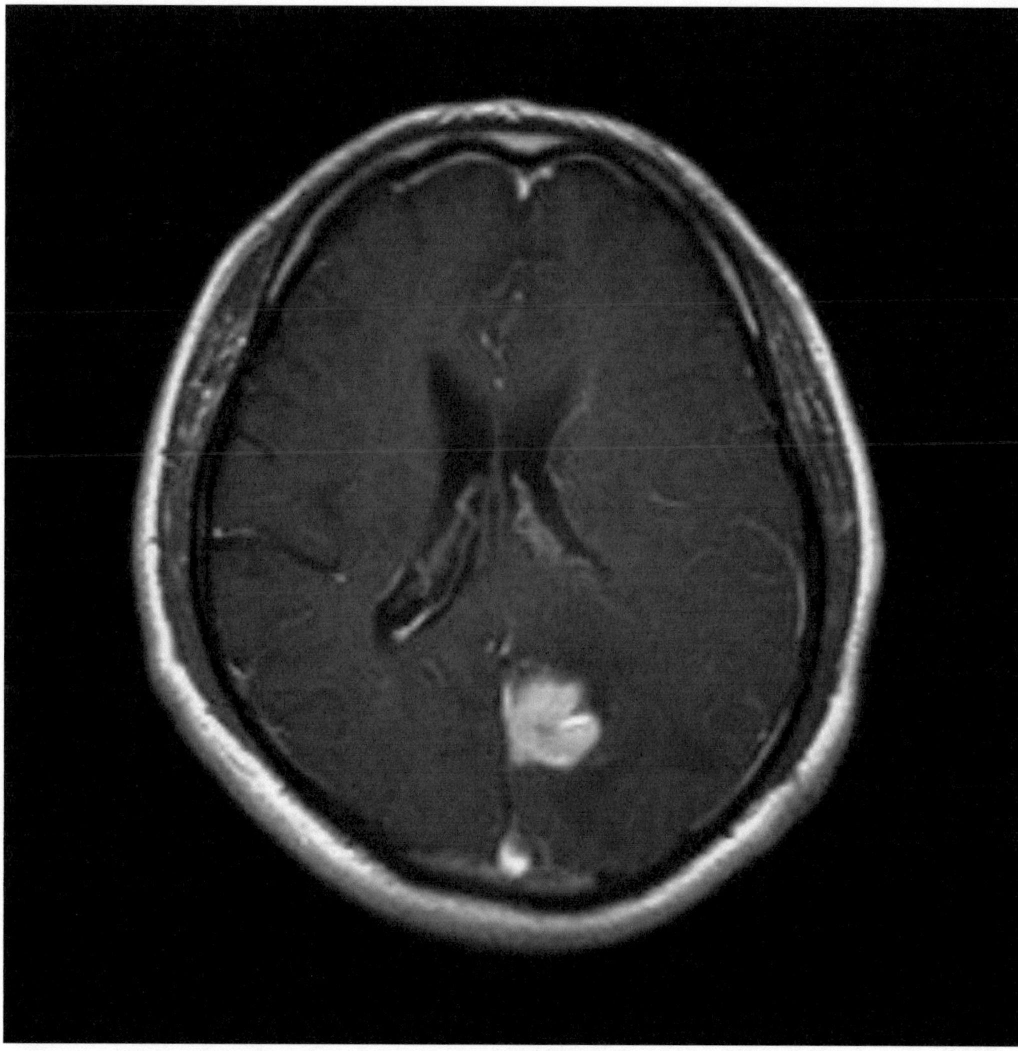

Fig. 6. Left occipital malignant lymphoma

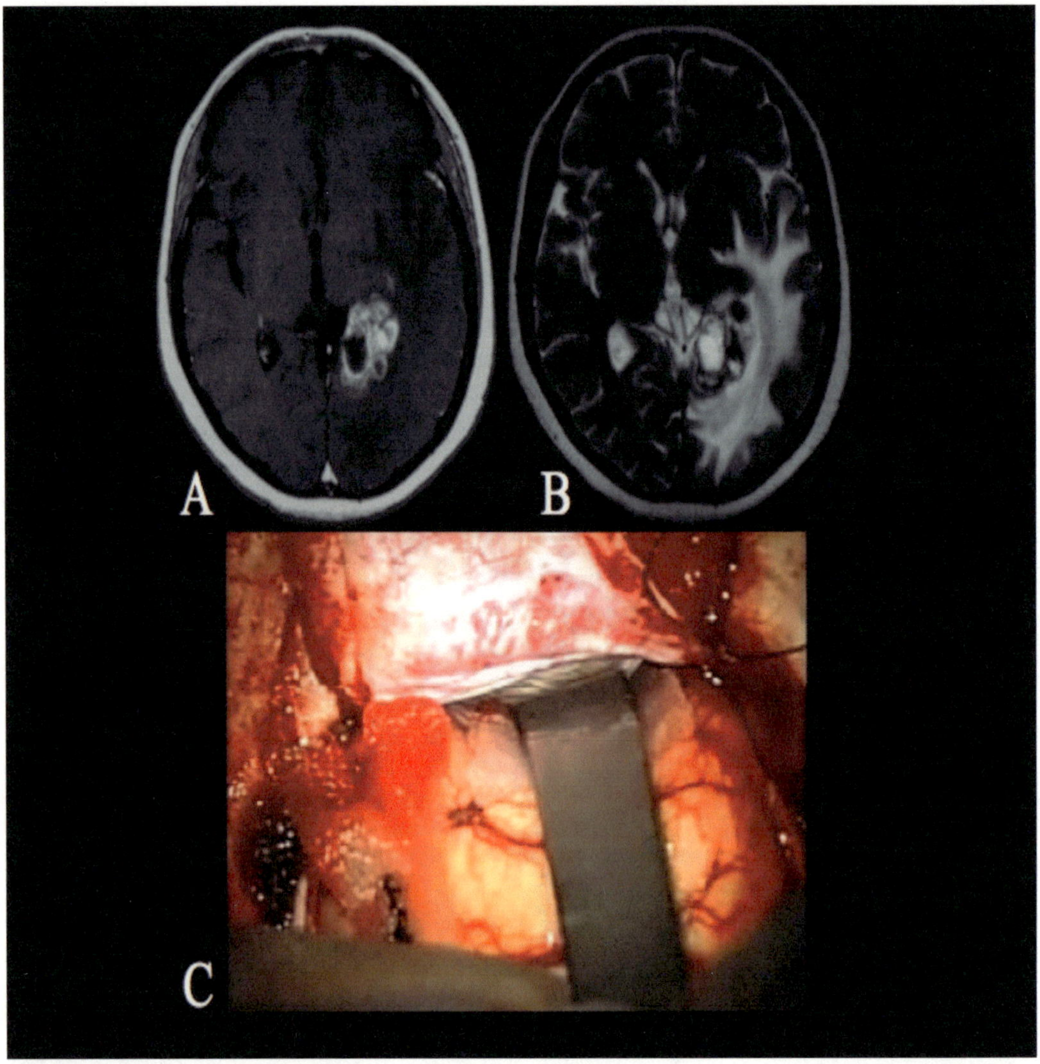

Fig. 7. Metastatic trigone tumor of the left trigone (A: T1-weighted image, B: T2-weighted image, and C: intraoperative view of the left occipital lobe)

2.8 Decision-making regarding the surgical approach for trigone meningiomas

The basic approach for a trigone meningioma is an occipital interhemispheric and transcortical one. A small or medium-sized tumor with a major blood supply from the posterior choroidal artery can be totally removed by this approach, even in patients with a tumor in the dominant hemisphere. A small or medium-sized trigone tumor supplied mainly by the anterior choroidal artery can also be removed via this single approach, although some blood loss can occur. For very large and vascular tumors fed equally by both the anterior and posterior choroidal arteries, an occipital interhemispheric and transcortical approach can be considered. For large vascular tumors in the non-dominant hemisphere fed mainly by the anterior choroidal arteries, an anterior temporal horn approach via an inferior temporo-occipital incision can be considered, although speech disturbance, epilepsy, or a visual field defect may occur. Large vascular tumors in the dominant ventricle fed mainly by the anterior choroidal arteries are potentially the most hazardous. Piecemeal resection of the tumor is mandatory when the occipital interhemispheric approach is used. Blood loss can be fatal, especially in pediatric patients. No single approach seems adequate for tumor excision. The anterior part of the tumor is first removed via an anterior temporal horn and trigone approach using an inferior temporo-occipital incision without incising the posterior middle temporal gyrus, and at second surgery, the posterior part of the tumor can be removed using an occipital interhemispheric approach. At the first operation, awake surgery by mapping cortical speech areas before reaching the tumor, may be useful to prevent speech and auditory comprehension deficits.

3. References

[1] Jelinek J, Smirniotopoulos JG, Parisi JE, Kanzer M (1990) Lateral ventricular neoplasms of the brain: differential diagnosis based on clinical, CT, and MR findings. Am J Roentgenol 155:365-372.

[2] Morrison G, Sobel DF, Kelley WM, Norman D (1984) Intraventricular mass lesions. Radiology 153:435-442.

[3] Al-Mefty O. 1991. Meningiomas. Raven Press, New York.

[4] Criscuolo GR, Symon L (1986) Intraventricular meningioma. A review of 10 cases of the National Hospital, Queen Square (1974-1985) with reference to the literature. Acta Neurochir (Wien) 83:83-91.

[5] Lyngdoh BT, Giri PJ, Behari S, Banerji D, Chhabra DK, Jain VK (2007) Intraventricular meningiomas: a surgical challenge. J Clin Neurosci 14:442-448.

[6] Bhatoe HS, Singh P, Dutta V (2006) Intraventricular meningiomas: a clinicopathological study and review. Neurosurg Focus 15;20:E9.

[7] Cushing H, Eisenhardt L. Meningiomas (1938) Their Classification, Regional Behavior, Life History and Surgical End Results. Springfield, IL: Charles C Thomas, pp 139-149.

[8] Couillard P, Karmi MZ, Abdelkader AM (1996) Microsurgical removal of an intraventricular meningioma with ultrasound guidance, and balloon dilation of operative corridors: case report and technical note. Surg Neurol 45:155-160.

[9] Fornari M, Savoiardo M, Morello G, Solero CL (1981) Meningiomas of the lateral ventricles. Neuroradiological and surgical considerations in 18 cases. J Neurosurg 54:64–74.

[10] Majós C, Cucurella G, Aguilera C, Coll S, Pons LC (1999) Intraventricular meningiomas: MR imaging and MR spectroscopic findings in two cases. Am J Neuroradiol 20:882-885.

[11] Mani RL, Hedgcock MW, Mass SI, Gilmor RL, Enzmann DR, Eisenberg RL (1978) Radiographic diagnosis of meningioma of the lateral ventricle. Review of 22 cases. J Neurosurg 49:249-255.

[12] Bertalanffy A, Roessler K, Koperek O, Gelpi E, Prayer D, Neuner M, Knosp E (2006) Intraventricular meningiomas: a report of 16 cases. Neurosurg Rev 29:30-35.

[13] Kempe LG, Blaylock R (1976) Lateral-trigonal intra-ventricular tumours. A new operative approach. Acta Neurochir (Wien) 35:233–242.

[14] Van Buren JM (1979) Anatomical study of a posterior cerebral lesion producing dyslexia. Neurosurgery 5:1–10.
[15] Hecaen H, de Ajuriaguerra J, David M (1952) Les Deficits fonctionnels apres lobectomie occipitale. Monatsschr Psychiatr Neurol 123:239 In French
[16] Schmidek HH, Sweet WH (1988) Operative Neurosurgical Techiniques. Indications, methods, and result. 2nd edit. Grune and Stratton. pp585
[17] Busch E (1939) Meningiomas of the lateral ventricles of the brain. Acta Chir Scand 82:282
[18] Gassel MM, Davies H (1961) Meningiomas in the lateral ventricles. Brain 84:605.
[19] Kempe LG (1968) Lateral intra-ventricular tumours (choroids plexus papilloma of the lateral ventricle), in Operative Neurosurgery, vol 1. Springer-Verlag, Berlin, pp 196–202
[20] Spencer DD, Collins WF (1982) Surgical management of lateral intra-ventricular tumours. In: Schmidek HH, Sweet WH (eds) Operative Neurosurgical Techniques: Indications, Methods, and Results, vol 1. Grune & Stratton, New York, pp 561–574
[21] Nagata S, Sasaki T (2005) Lateral trans-sulcal approach to asymptomatic trigonal meningiomas with correlative microsurgical anatomy: Technical case report. Neurosurgery 56:438.
[22] Nishizaki T, Ikeda N, Nakano S, Okamura T, Abiko S (2009) Occipital inter-hemispheric approach for lateral ventricular trigone meningioma. Acta Neurochir. 151: 1717-1721.